ORTHOPEDIC CLINICS OF NORTH AMERICA

www.orthopedic.theclinics.com

Orthopedic Urgencies and Emergencies

January 2022 • Volume 53 • Number 1

ELSEVIER

1600 John F. Kennedy Boulevard • Suite 1800 • Philadelphia, Pennsylvania, 19103-2899.

http://www.orthopedic.theclinics.com

ORTHOPEDIC CLINICS OF NORTH AMERICA Volume 53, Number 1
January 2022 ISSN 0030-5898, ISBN-13: 978-0-323-84967-8

Editor: Lauren Boyle
Developmental Editor: Ann Gielou Posedio

Orthopedic Clinics of North America (ISSN 0030-5898) is published quarterly by Elsevier Inc., 360 Park Avenue South, New York, NY 10010-1710. Months of issue are January, April, July, and October. Business and Editorial Offices: 1600 John F. Kennedy Blvd., Suite 1800, Philadelphia, PA 19103-2899. Customer Service Office: 3251 Riverport Lane, Maryland Heights, MO 63043. Periodicals postage paid at New York, NY and additional mailing offices. Subscription prices are $354.00 per year for (US individuals), $1,033.00 per year for (US institutions), $420.00 per year (Canadian individuals), $1,064.00 per year (Canadian institutions), $486.00 per year (international individuals), $1,064.00 per year (international institutions), $100.00 per year (US students), $100.00 per year for (Canadian students), $220.00 per year for (international students). Foreign air speed delivery is included in all *Clinics* subscription prices. All prices are subject to change without notice. **POSTMASTER:** Send change of address to *Orthopedic Clinics of North America*, **Elsevier Health Sciences Division, Subscription Customer Service, 3251 Riverport Lane, Maryland Heights, MO 63043. Customer Service (orders, claims, online, change of address): Elsevier Health Sciences Division, Subscription Customer Service, 3251 Riverport Lane, Maryland Heights, MO 63043. Tel: 1-800-654-2452 (U.S. and Canada); 314-447-8871 (outside U.S. and Canada). Fax: 314-447-8029. E-mail:** journalscustomerservice-usa@elsevier.com **(for print support);** journalsonlinesupport-usa@elsevier.com **(for online support).**

Reprints. For copies of 100 or more, of articles in this publication, please contact the Commercial Reprints Department, Elsevier Inc., 360 Park Avenue South, New York, NY 10010-1710. Tel.: 212-633-3874; Fax: 212-633-3820; E-mail: reprints@elsevier.com.

Orthopedic Clinics of North America is covered in *MEDLINE/PubMed* (*Index Medicus*), *Cinahl, Excerpta Medica,* and *Cumulative Index to Nursing and Allied Health Literature.*

EDITORIAL BOARD

CONTRIBUTORS

EDITOR

FREDERICK M. AZAR, MD
Professor, Department of Orthopaedic
Surgery and Biomedical Engineering,
University of Tennessee Campbell Clinic,
Memphis, Tennessee, USA

AUTHORS

MICHAEL H. AMINI, MD
Shoulder and Elbow Surgery, The CORE
Institute, Phoenix, Arizona, USA

CHARLES LOWRY BARNES, MD
Chairman, Department of Orthopedic
Surgery, University of Arkansas for Medical
Sciences, Little Rock, Arkansas, USA

CHAD CAMPION, MD
Norton Leatherman Spine Center, Louisville,
Kentucky, USA

LEAH Y. CARREON, MD, MSc
Norton Leatherman Spine Center, Louisville,
Kentucky, USA

JEFFREY S. CHEN, MD
Department of Orthopedic Surgery, NYU
Langone Orthopedic Hospital, NYU Langone
Health, New York, New York, USA

CHRISTOPHER T. COSGROVE, MD
Orthopaedic Surgery Department, Campbell
Clinic Orthopaedics, University of Tennessee
Health Science Center, Memphis, Tennessee,
USA

CHARLES H. CRAWFORD III, MD
Norton Leatherman Spine Center,
Department of Orthopaedic Surgery,
University of Louisville School of Medicine,
Louisville, Kentucky, USA

SHAUNETTE DAVEY, DO, FAAOS
Pediatric Orthopaedic Fellow, Children's
Healthcare of Atlanta, Atlanta, Georgia, USA

JOHN R. DIMAR II, MD
Norton Leatherman Spine Center, University
of Louisville School of Medicine, Department
of Orthopaedic Surgery, Louisville, Kentucky,
USA

MLADEN DJURASOVIC, MD
Norton Leatherman Spine Center, Louisville,
Kentucky, USA

TRAVIS B. EASON, MD
Orthopaedic Surgery Department, Campbell
Clinic Orthopaedics, University of Tennessee
Health Science Center, Memphis, Tennessee,
USA

JOHN J. FELDMAN, MD
Department of Orthopaedic Surgery, Jersey
City Medical Center/Saint Barnabas Medical
Center-RWJ Barbabas Health, Jersey City,
New Jersey, USA

TUESDAY FISHER, MD
Assistant Professor, Department of Surgery,
Uniformed Services University of the Health
Sciences, Bethesda, Maryland, USA

STEVEN D. GLASSMAN, MD
Norton Leatherman Spine Center,
Department of Orthopaedic Surgery,
University of Louisville School of Medicine,
Louisville, Kentucky, USA

JEFFREY L. GUM, MD
Norton Leatherman Spine Center, Louisville,
Kentucky, USA

ERICK M. HEIMAN, DO
Department of Orthopaedic Surgery, Jersey City Medical Center/Saint Barnabas Medical Center-RWJ Barbabas Health, Jersey City, New Jersey, USA

LISA C. HOWARD, MD, MHSc, FRCSC
Orthopaedic Surgeon, Lower Limb Reconstruction, Department of Orthopaedics, University of British Columbia, Department of Orthopaedics, Diamond Health Care Centre, Complex Joint Clinic, Vancouver, British Columbia, Canada

JACLYN M. JANKOWSKI, DO
Department of Orthopaedic Surgery, Jersey City Medical Center/Saint Barnabas Medical Center-RWJ Barbabas Health, Jersey City, New Jersey, USA

BASSAM A. MASRI, MD, FRCSC
Department of Orthopaedics, Diamond Health Care Centre, Complex Joint Clinic, Professor of Orthopaedics, University of British Columbia, Vancouver, British Columbia, Canada; Head of Orthopaedics, Vancouver Acute Health Services

SIMON C. MEARS, MD, PhD
Professor, Department of Orthopedic Surgery, University of Arkansas for Medical Sciences, Little Rock, Arkansas, USA

WILLIAM M. MIHALKO, MD, PhD
Orthopaedic Surgery Department, Campbell Clinic Orthopaedics, University of Tennessee Health Science Center, Memphis, Tennessee, USA

PETER N. MITTWEDE, MD, PhD
Department of Orthopaedic Surgery, University of Pittsburgh, Pittsburgh, Pennsylvania, USA

CHRISTOPHER D. MURAWSKI, MD
Department of Orthopaedic Surgery, University of Pittsburgh, Pittsburgh, Pennsylvania, USA

NAVEED NABIZADEH, MD
Norton Leatherman Spine Center, Louisville, Kentucky, USA

MICHAEL E. NEUFELD, MD, MSc, FRCSC
Orthopaedic Surgeon, Lower Limb Reconstruction, Department of Orthopaedics, University of British Columbia, Department of Orthopaedics, Diamond Health Care Centre, Complex Joint Clinic, Vancouver, British Columbia, Canada

ROBERT V. O'TOOLE, MD
Division Head, Orthopaedic Traumatology, R Adams Cowley Shock Trauma Center, University of Maryland School of Medicine, Baltimore, Maryland, USA

KARAN M. PATEL, BA
Medical Student, University of Arkansas for Medical Sciences, Little Rock, Arkansas, USA

MIDHAT PATEL, MD
Department of Orthopedics, University of Arizona College of Medicine – Phoenix, Phoenix, Arizona, USA

M. LUCIUS POMERANTZ, MD, FAAOS
Orthopedic Surgeon, Hand/Upper Extremity Specialist, Synergy Orthopedic Specialists, Inc, Health Sciences Assistant Clinical Professor (Non-Salaried), Orthopedic Surgery, University of California, San Diego, San Diego, California, USA

BRIAN A. SCHNEIDERMAN, MD
Assistant Professor, Department of Orthopaedics, Loma Linda University Health, Loma Linda, California, USA

TIM SCHRADER, MD
Chief of Hip Preservation, Children's Healthcare of Atlanta, Atlanta, Georgia, USA

ARESH SEPEHRI, MD, MSc
Department of Orthopaedics, University of British Columbia, Vancouver, British Columbia, Canada

JEFFREY B. STAMBOUGH, MD
Assistant Professor, Department of Orthopedic Surgery, University of Arkansas for Medical Sciences, Little Rock, Arkansas, USA

MATTHEW W.J. STREET, MBChB, MMSc, FRACS
Clinical Fellow, Lower Limb Reconstruction, Department of Orthopaedics, University of

British Columbia, Department of
Orthopaedics, Diamond Health Care Centre,
Complex Joint Clinic, Vancouver, British
Columbia, Canada

BENJAMIN M. STRONACH, MS, MD
Associate Professor, Department of
Orthopedic Surgery, University of Arkansas for
Medical Sciences, Little Rock, Arkansas, USA

IVAN S. TARKIN, MD
Professor and Chief of Trauma, Department of
Orthopaedic Surgery, University of Pittsburgh,
Pittsburgh, Pennsylvania, USA

NIRMAL C. TEJWANI, MD
Professor, Department of Orthopedic
Surgery, NYU Langone Orthopedic Hospital,
NYU Langone Health, New York, New York,
USA

RICHARD S. YOON, MD
Director of Orthopaedic Research,
Department of Orthopaedic Surgery, Jersey
City Medical Center/Saint Barnabas Medical
Center-RWJ Barbabas Health, Jersey City,
New Jersey, USA

CONTENTS

Symptomatic postoperative epidural hematomas are rare, with an incidence of
0.10% to 0.69%. Risk factors have varied in the literature, but multiple studies
have reported advanced age, preoperative or postoperative coagulopathy,
and multilevel laminectomy as risk factors for hematoma. The role of pharmacologic anticoagulation after spine surgery remains unclear, but multiple
studies suggest it can be done safely with a low risk of epidural hematoma. Prophylactic suction drains have not been found to lower hematoma incidence.
Most symptomatic postoperative epidural hematomas present within the first
24 to 48 hours after surgery but can present later. Diagnosis of a symptomatic
hematoma requires correlation of clinical signs and symptoms with a compressive hematoma on MRI. Patients will usually first complain of a marked increase
in axial pain, followed by radicular symptoms in the extremities, followed by
motor weakness and sphincter dysfunction. An MRI should be obtained emergently, and if it confirms a compressive hematoma, surgical evacuation should
be carried out as quickly as possible. The prognosis for neurologic improvement after evacuation depends on the time delay and the degree of neurologic
impairment before evacuation.

ORTHOPEDIC URGENCIES AND EMERGENCIES

DEDICATION

It is with deep appreciation and admiration that we dedicate this issue to Kay C. Daugherty, who served as Senior Medical Editor at the Campbell Foundation for over 43 years. In addition to editing and overseeing innumerable publications produced by the Campbell Clinic physicians, Kay also was instrumental in the publication of *Orthopedic Clinics of North America*, serving as the editorial manager over the last 5 years. Her writing and editorial expertise will remain the gold standard for medical editing throughout the publishing community, and her loyal service to our organization as well as many others in our field will continue to impact orthopedic surgeons worldwide.

Orthop Clin N Am 53 (2022) xv
https://doi.org/10.1016/j.ocl.2021.11.001
0030-5898/22/© 2021 Published by Elsevier Inc.

PREFACE

Trauma to or infection of any part of the musculo-skeletal system, in general, falls under the category of urgent or emergent orthopedic care. Timing and immediacy of treatment depend on the severity of injury, which can range from minor, such as a strain or a sprain, to critical, when survival of the limb or the patient is uncertain. This issue reviews injuries and conditions that require urgent attention to preserve life, limb, and functional outcomes.

Dr Matthew Street and colleagues provide a review of vascular injuries associated with hip and knee arthroplasty. Although such injuries are rare, they can result in devastating outcomes. These authors discuss the intraoperative mechanisms of these injuries, identify the risk factors involved, and describe ways to avoid or manage this complication. Another complication that is increasing with the rise in total joint arthroplasties is sepsis. Dr Karan Patel and colleagues review periprosthetic joint infections that can lead to sepsis after total joint arthroplasty. Sepsis is a life-threatening organ dysfunction caused by dysregulation of host response from an infection. The authors describe the appropriate treatment of sepsis, with and without PJI, as these patients are at high risk for mortality. Acute compartment syndrome, another dreaded complication after total joint surgery, is the focus of a discussion by Dr Areh Sepehri and colleagues. Early diagnosis and prompt definitive management are paramount in preventing the significant morbidity associated with this complication. This review article includes how to identify compartment syndrome after surgery given the immediate postoperative pain patients experience and possible risk factors involved. To follow, Drs Eason, Cosgrove, and Mihalko present the epidemiology, classification, diagnosis, and treatment of necrotizing soft-tissue infection after hip arthroplasty. These infections are associated with a high mortality, and diagnosis and treatment must be expeditious.

Dr Schneiderman and Dr O'Toole review acute compartment syndrome after tibial plateau fractures. These fractures already carry a high risk of this complication. The authors discuss demographic, clinical, and radiographic factors associated with the development of compartment syndrome in this scenario. They note that

management includes emergent compartment decompression, but fracture fixation often complicates the treatment course, and deep surgical site infection is common.

Unstable slipped capital femoral epiphysis is a well-recognized disorder in the pediatric and adolescent population that requires urgent care. This disease carries potential long-term sequelae that may result in osteonecrosis and permanently affect hip function. Drs Davey, Fisher, and Schrader provide a succinct overview of this disease process, the incidence and demographic features, as well as the controversies surrounding treatment.

Necrotizing fasciitis, as in other limbs, is a difficult-to-treat infection in hand and wrist injuries. The review by Dr Lucius Pomerantz describes its presentation, which is often difficult to recognize, and the speed of spread. Prompt surgical treatment with the use of a multidisciplinary team is necessary to optimize outcomes, although they note that there is still high mortality and morbidity reported.

An absolute orthopedic emergency in the upper extremity is scapulothoracic dissociation, a rare but devastating injury. Dr Heiman and colleagues present a review of the mechanism of injury, physical examination, radiographic parameters, evaluation of ischemia, and management focused on resuscitation. A lesser injury in the shoulder, but one that also can have long-term consequences, is acute rotator cuff tear. Drs Patel and Amini describe treatment options for partial and full-thickness tears, noting that better outcomes can be expected if treatment is rendered within 4 months of injury.

In the foot and ankle, compartment syndrome is an uncommon but potentially devastating condition that requires emergent recognition and treatment. Drs Chen and Tejwani describe how its presentation is often less clear than compartment syndrome in other limb compartments and requires a low threshold for direct measurement of compartment pressure. Controversy surrounds the most effective treatment, and both immediate surgical treatment and delayed treatment can result in significant and long-term sequelae. Drs Garkin, Murawki, and Mittwede then present a review of temporizing procedures for acute

Orthop Clin N Am 53 (2022) xvii–xviii
https://doi.org/10.1016/j.ocl.2021.10.001

traumatic foot and ankle injuries. Factors such as complexity of injury, amount of soft tissue damage, and patient's medical history affect treatment type and whether to proceed with staged or definitive treatment.

Neurologic deficits, especially in spine injuries, are considered orthopedic emergencies. Dr Nabizadeh and colleagues provide a systematic review of neurologic deficits in patients with pyogenic spondylodiscitis. Prompt diagnosis and surgical intervention are associated with a greater chance of improvement in status in these patients. Another emergent condition that can cause neurologic compromise in the spine is postoperative epidural hematoma. Drs Djurasovic and colleagues provide a review of the incidence, risk factors, presentation, and diagnosis of compressive hematoma. MRI and surgical evacuation must be carried out as quickly as possible, as prognosis for improvement depends on time delay and the degree of neurologic impairment by the time of recognition.

We would like to thank the authors for their excellent contributions to this issue and hope that these review articles will be beneficial to orthopedists in identifying and treating orthopedic emergencies.

Frederick M. Azar, MD
Professor, Department of Orthopaedic Surgery &
Biomedical Engineering
University of Tennessee–Campbell Clinic
1211 Union Avenue, Suite 510
Memphis, TN 38104, USA

E-mail address:
fazar@campbellclinic.com

Knee and Hip Reconstruction

Vascular Injuries During Hip and Knee Replacement

Matthew W.J. Street, MBChB, MMSc, FRACS[a,b,*], Lisa C. Howard, MD, MHSc, FRCSC[a,b],
Michael E. Neufeld, MD, MSc, FRCSC[a,b], Bassam A. Masri, MD, FRCSC[b,c,d]

KEYWORDS

- Hip replacement • Knee replacement • Vascular injury • Complications

KEY POINTS

- The incidence of vascular injury during total hip arthroplasty is 0.04% to 0.1%. Direct injury to the external iliac artery or the common femoral artery is the most common mechanism of injury.
- The incidence of vascular injury during total knee arthroplasty is 0.057% to 0.19%. Indirect injury to the popliteal artery, causing intimal tear, thrombus, and ischemia, is most common, although direct vascular injuries can occur.
- Revision surgery is a major risk factor for vascular injury.
- Immediate preoperative and postoperative examination of vascular status is recommended.
- Early diagnosis and intervention are critical to avoid poor outcomes.

INTRODUCTION

Vascular injuries during hip and knee replacement are rare but potentially devastating. They may result in loss of life or limb and commonly result in litigation against the surgeon.

The following review aims to provide insight into this Orthopedic emergency and ultimately to help improve outcomes for patients. The authors highlight the following:

- The epidemiology of vascular injuries, including identifying high-risk patients who may require further preoperative workup.
- Relevant vascular anatomy, mechanisms of injury, and techniques to avoid injury to the vessels.
- The presentation and diagnosis of vascular injuries associated with hip and knee replacement.
- The management and outcomes of vascular injuries, with guidance to avoid

further complications through timely diagnosis and intervention.

A sound knowledge of relevant vascular anatomy, with thorough preoperative assessment and careful operative technique, may help avoid these dreaded complications. When they do occur, early diagnosis via routine postoperative vascular examination may lead to improved outcomes with early intervention.

THE HIP

Incidence

Vascular injury during primary total hip arthroplasty is rare. Historically, the incidence was reported at 0.25%.[1] However, recent large studies report an incidence of 0.04% to 0.1%.[2–6] The incidence in revision surgery has been reported as 0.05% to 0.2%.[2,4,5]

The external iliac and common femoral vessels are the most commonly injured vessels during total hip arthroplasty.[7,8]

[a] Lower Limb Reconstruction, Department of Orthopaedics, University of British Columbia, Vancouver, British Columbia, Canada; [b] Department of Orthopaedics, Diamond Health Care Centre, Complex Joint Clinic, 3rd Floor, 2775 Laurel Street, Vancouver, British Columbia V5Z 1M9, Canada; [c] University of British Columbia, Vancouver, British Columbia, Canada; [d] Vancouver Acute Health Services
* Corresponding author. Department of Orthopaedics, Diamond Health Care Centre, Complex Joint Clinic, 3rd Floor, 2775 Laurel Street, Vancouver, British Columbia V5Z 1M9, Canada.
E-mail address: matthewstreet_77@hotmail.com

Orthop Clin N Am 53 (2022) 1–12
https://doi.org/10.1016/j.ocl.2021.08.009

Risk Factors

Multiple risk factors have been described for vascular injury during total hip arthroplasty. The most significant risk factor for vascular injury is revision surgery.[4–7,9,10] Abularrage and colleagues[4] found an incidence of 0.2% during revision surgery (4/2033) compared with 0.04% in primary surgery (6/13,494). Similarly, Troutman and colleagues[5] found an increased risk of 0.12% in revision surgery (3/2529) compared with 0.09% in primary surgery (9/10,293). Avisar and colleagues[6] reported 2 vascular complications out of 1601 total hips, both occurring in revision operations. Shoenfeld and colleagues[7] presented 68 cases of vascular injury, of which 39% occurred during revision surgery. Fukunishi and colleagues[11] carried out computed tomography (CT) angiograms on complex total hip arthroplasty patients and found vascular proliferation and reduced distance of major vessels from the acetabulum in revision cases, as well as those with proximally migrated femurs and ankylosed hips. The risk of vascular injury when revising a medially migrated acetabular component, along with the risk associated with acetabular screws and antiprotrusio cages, has been well reported.[7,12–14] Revision for infection has also been identified as a risk for vascular injury.[9,15]

Higher vascular complications have also been reported in women, left-sided surgeries, and the African American population.[4,7,9,10] Kawasaki and colleagues[16] performed CT angiograms on 200 normal hips and found the major vessels were closer to the acetabulum in women and on the left side. They also found that in older patients the vessels were more tortuous and closer to the acetabulum.

Preexisting atherosclerosis or previous vascular intervention is a risk factor for indirect injury and thrombosis. Alshameeri and colleagues[10] identified 4 of 18 patients with thrombotic lesions that had underlying peripheral vascular disease. They identified a further 4 patients who had a synthetic bypass graft occlusion during surgery.

Anatomy

The external iliac and common femoral arteries are the most commonly injured vessels during total hip arthroplasty.[3,7,10]

The common iliac artery bifurcates into the internal iliac artery and external iliac artery at the L5/S1 disc level. The external iliac artery and vein continue along the inner table of the pelvis, relatively tethered by the pelvic peritoneum and branching nutrient vessels,[17] and becomes the common femoral artery as it passes beneath the inguinal ligament (Fig. 1).

The common femoral artery continues anterior and medial to the hip capsule and the anterior wall of the acetabulum. It is separated from the acetabulum only by the capsule and psoas muscle. On the surface of the psoas, the femoral vein lies medial to the common femoral artery, and the femoral nerve lies lateral. The distance of this important vascular pedicle from the acetabulum has been characterized via cadaver and CT angiogram studies. Feugier and colleagues[17] report an average of 8 mm from the anterior cortex to the vessels at the mid acetabulum level. Fukunishi and colleagues[11] examined preoperative CT angiograms in complex primary and revision hips, finding an average distance of 12 mm from the anterior acetabulum to the vessels in primary hips, and 16 mm in revision hips. The increased distance in revision hips is likely due to scar tissue and capsular thickening following primary total hip arthroplasty. However, this increased distance may not imply a reduced risk, as revision surgery often necessitates further debridement and more forceful retraction to gain exposure, and the vessels are likely more tethered.

The associated external iliac/common femoral vein lies more medially and is less commonly injured.[7]

The common femoral artery gives off the profunda femoris artery before continuing as the superficial femoral artery in the subsartorial canal. The profunda femoris artery and its large perforator branches may be injured during distal and posterior dissection around the femur and placement of cerclage cables/wires.

The obturator artery arises from the anterior trunk of the internal iliac artery and passes over the quadrilateral surface of the acetabulum,

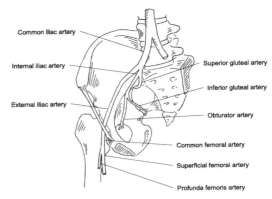

Fig. 1. Arterial anatomy of the hip.

separated from bone by the thin obturator internus muscle. It may lie as close as 2 mm to the bony surface at the inferior portion of the acetabulum.[18]

Posteriorly, the superior gluteal artery arises from the posterior trunk of the internal iliac artery and passes through the superior aspect of the greater sciatic notch. The inferior gluteal artery arises from the anterior trunk of the internal iliac artery and passes over the ischial spine. The superior gluteal artery lies an average of 5 mm from bone and the inferior gluteal artery an average of 6 mm from bone; however, both gluteal arteries are surrounded by loose areolar tissue, providing them some degree of mobility and protection and making injury less common.[19]

The Safe Quadrants

The acetabular quadrants for safe screw placement were described by Wasielewski and colleagues[20] to avoid the at-risk vessels, particularly the external iliac/common femoral vessels.

A line is visualized from the anterior superior iliac spine to the ischium, through the center of the acetabulum. Both of these landmarks are easily palpated intraoperatively. A line is visualized perpendicular to this through the center of the acetabulum, thus dividing the acetabulum into 4 quadrants: posterosuperior, posteroinferior, anteroinferior, and anterosuperior (Fig. 2).

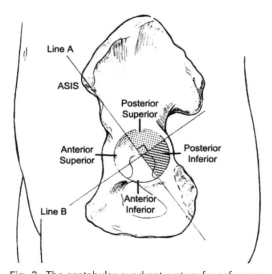

Fig. 2. The acetabular quadrant system for safe screw insertion. (*From* Wasielewski RC et al. Acetabular anatomy and the transacetabular fixation of screws in total hip arthroplasty. J Bone Joint Surg Am 1990;72:501-8, with permission.)

The posterosuperior and posteroinferior quadrants are generally considered safe zones for screw placement, providing adequate bone stock for fixation with limited risk to neurovascular structures.

The posterosuperior quadrant provides the best corridor for screw fixation, with screw lengths of 60 mm or greater when directed toward the sacroiliac joint.[17] Care must be taken to avoid the superior gluteal neurovascular bundle within the greater sciatic notch in more posteriorly directed screws; however, these vessels lie off the bone within mobile areolar tissue, providing some degree of protection. Nevertheless, the authors recommend that a finger be gently placed on the bone in the greater sciatic notch when a drill bit is directed in that direction, to avoid plunging and possible vascular injury.

The posteroinferior quadrant provides bone stock for screws up to 35 mm.[17] Care must be taken to avoid the inferior gluteal and pudendal vessels; however, these are similarly mobile and thus relatively protected.[17] During a posterior approach, the posterior wall can similarly be carefully palpated and the tip of a depth gauge or screw can often be felt to ensure appropriate screw length and clearance from neurovascular structures.

It is important to note that in both posterior quadrants the central portion should be avoided, as the trajectory puts the obturator vessels deep to the quadrilateral plate in danger, and the obturator internus muscle provides minimal protection.[17]

The anterosuperior and anteroinferior quadrants are both considered unsafe.

A drill or screw placed in the anterosuperior quadrant would be directed through the thin anterior wall toward the tethered external iliac/common femoral vessels. These vessels were injured with 75% of screws placed in this quadrant in 1 cadaver study.[17]

A drill or screw in the anteroinferior quadrant puts the obturator pedicle at high risk for injury.

Meldrum and Lance Johansen[21] investigated the safety of the quadrant system in revision scenarios using a cadaveric model. They found the quadrant system held true when using a jumbo cup, with no vascular insults in the posterosuperior or posteroinferior quadrants. When reconstructing with a high hip center, however, the center and anterior halves of the posterosuperior quadrant were unsafe, risking injury to the external iliac or obturator vessels. If using cages, they noted the posterosuperior extra-acetabular screws were safe as long as they were directed perpendicular to the ilium. If the construct was retroverted, these screws became unsafe. If using ischial screw fixation, they found 33% of screws injured the pudendal vessels. It is therefore important to proceed with caution when drilling and to constantly palpate to make sure that the far cortex is not perforated.

Mechanism of Injury

Direct injury remains the most common mechanism of vascular injury during total hip arthroplasty, in contrast to indirect injury during total knee arthroplasty.[3,10] Nachbur and colleagues[1] described the 4 main mechanisms of injury:

- Direct vascular perforation by the tip of a Hohmann retractor
- Direct laceration during instrumentation/implantation
- Overextension of atherosclerotic arteries causing intimal injury and subsequent thrombus formation
- Thrombosis secondary to excessive heat produced by cement polymerization.

Shoenfeld and colleagues[7] reported on 68 cases, with 44% cement-related injuries, 18% retractor related, 10% due to excessive traction on vessels, 7% related to medial cup migration, 3% due to reaming injury, 1% osteotome injury, and 16% unknown.

Excessive intrapelvic cement, in particular, any sharp cement spiculae, may cause injury to intrapelvic vessels. This may occur by mechanical pressure or gradual erosion of vessels over sharp spiculae, or secondary to the heat-produced and resultant thrombosis during cement polymerization.[1,9]

With the transition to cementless acetabular implants, cement-related vascular complications are now less common. However, vascular injuries related to drill and screw penetration and, in particular, acetabular revision, are more commonly reported.[20,22–24] During acetabular revision, vascular injury may occur during debridement and retractor placement in a more difficult exposure, during implant removal or reaming, particularly in cases with a medialized acetabular component or deficient medial wall, or during drilling/screw placement during cup or augment fixation.

Safe Retractor Placement

Direct vascular injury from aberrant placement of retractors is a common mechanism of injury.[1,7] Shubert and colleagues[25] studied preoperative CTs and cadavers to determine safe placement of the anterior acetabular retractor. They identified the anterior inferior iliac spine as the safest position for anterior acetabular retractor placement, being on average 2.65 cm from the common femoral vessels. With more inferior retractor placement, the distance to the common femoral vessels was reduced, being only an average of 0.95 cm away in the anteroinferior position.

Care should be taken in anterior Hohmann placement, positioning the retractor between bone and capsule in the anterosuperior portion of the anterior wall (**Fig. 3**).

The obturator vessels may also be damaged during placement of an inferior acetabular retractor. Care should be taken here to remain against bone and avoid plunging with the sharp tip of the Hohmann.

The posterior retractor poses more risk to the sciatic nerve than the gluteal vessels. Nonetheless, this retractor should be placed with care between the capsule and the posterior wall of the acetabulum.

Preoperative Assessment

Prevention of vascular injury begins in the clinic, with a thorough history and examination. A vascular assessment should be carried out whenever planning for total hip arthroplasty.

History should query symptoms of claudication or ischemic limb pain. History of lower limb angioplasty or bypass surgery should be identified, along with any other vascular procedures, such as coronary artery stenting/bypass, carotid endarterectomy, aortic aneurysm repair. A history of smoking, diabetes, hypertension, dyslipidemia, and cardiovascular or cerebrovascular disease will allow a risk assessment for associated peripheral vascular disease.

Examination of the lower limb should identify changes of chronic ischemia, including skin discoloration, absence of hair, dystrophic nail changes, and skin ulceration. The pedal pulses should be examined and compared with the contralateral side.

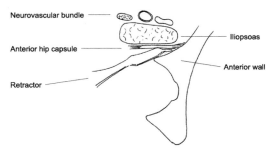

Fig. 3. Safe placement of the anterior acetabular retractor.

Radiographs should be examined for vessel calcification.

If any concerns for vascular disease or insufficiency exist, then ankle brachial indices (ABI) can be obtained. An ABI of less than 0.9 suggests arterial disease, whereas an ABI of less than 0.5 indicates severe disease.

A referral for vascular consultation and consideration of further imaging and potential intervention has been suggested in patients with significant risk identified on history and examination, in particular, if they have absent or markedly attenuated pedal pulses.[2]

Revision for medial cup migration and/or removal of intrapelvic cement has been widely reported as high risk for vascular injury.[7,12–14,26,27] In these cases, preoperative CT angiography and review with a vascular surgeon is indicated, and consideration should be made for a retroperitoneal approach for visualization and protection of the external iliac vessels during component removal.

Presentation and Management

Vascular injuries associated with total hip arthroplasty most commonly present as acute intraoperative hemorrhage from direct vessel injury.[1,3,6,10,12] Alshameeri and colleagues[10] found this accounted for 53% of cases in their systematic review. Intraoperative diagnosis of direct vascular injury is often obvious and necessitates emergent vascular intervention.

The next most prevalent presentation is ischemia secondary to thrombus formation.[3,10] The diagnosis with this presentation can be more challenging, leading to delays in diagnosis and treatment.[2,5] Calligaro and colleagues[2] found that half of patients presenting with ischemia were not diagnosed until postoperative day 1 to 3. Thus, it must be considered part of every total hip replacement to check the patient's pedal pulses preoperatively and immediately postoperatively. If these are absent or significantly reduced compared with the preoperative assessment, then emergent vascular consultation and CT angiogram should be sought.

Finally, patients may present late with sequelae of a pseudoaneurysm formation. A pseudoaneurysm may form after less severe vascular injury, causing slow bleeding and delayed symptoms. They may present in 3 ways: pressure-related pain in the hip, ischemic-related limb pain owing to impaired blood flow or distal microemboli, or severe bleeding during a later revision.[9] Alshameeri and colleagues[10] reported a delayed diagnosis

of greater than 1 month to greater than 1 year for pseudoaneurysms. Shoenfeld and colleagues[7] reported a mean delay to diagnosis of 29 months, and Bach and colleagues[28] reported a case diagnosed 14 years after the primary procedure.

As most vascular injuries during total hip arthroplasty occur by direct laceration, causing intraoperative hemorrhage, the mainstay of treatment is concurrent open vascular surgery.[2,3,5,10] During these situations, maintaining composure and communicating efficiently with all team members are of paramount importance. Alerting the anesthesia team is important to facilitate proper hemodynamic control and blood products when necessary. An emergent vascular surgery consultation is crucial with major vessel injury.

As with any vascular injury, gaining wide exposure and proximal control, when possible, are the initial principles of management. After exposure, control of minor vessels with direct pressure, cautery, vascular clips, or suture ligation can be considered. Hemostatic agents can also be considered. For major vessel injury, a partial laceration may be addressed by primary repair or patch angioplasty, whereas a complete laceration may occasionally be addressed by end-to-end anastomosis, but more frequently requires an interposition graft or bypass.[2]

Endovascular procedures are appealing and have been used more frequently in recent reports[5,10]; however, application of these techniques is limited in the setting of acute hemorrhage during total hip arthroplasty, as the lateral positioning, sterile field, and metal prostheses limit endovascular access and the use of fluoroscopy.[29] Endovascular intervention is more appropriately used for those patients diagnosed postoperatively with ischemia or pseudoaneurysm.[5] Occasionally, endovascular intervention may be considered when the source of bleeding cannot be identified or managed with initial open exploration. Mavrogenis and colleagues[30] reviewed 31 patients treated with embolization following elective orthopedic procedures and found the treatment was most effective for branch vessels/noncritical axial vessels, most commonly the superior gluteal vessels.

Outcomes

Vascular injuries can be associated with severe complications, including death and loss of limb.[4,7–10] Shoenfeld and colleagues[7] reported a mortality of 7% and amputation rate of 19% among 68 patients. Lazarides and colleagues[8] reported 9% mortality and 12% amputation rates along with 17% having permanent disability owing to ischemia. Alshameeri and colleagues[10] reported a 7.3% mortality, 1.6% amputation, and 7.3% persistent ischemia.

A delay to diagnosis is associated with inferior outcomes. Abularrage and colleagues[4] reported no amputations when vascular injury was diagnosed in the first 5 days compared with a 25% amputation rate when diagnosed after 5 days. Calligaro and colleagues[2] reported no deaths or amputations in their series; however, when diagnosis was delayed, more patients required fasciotomy and suffered from foot drop. This underscores the importance of an immediate postoperative vascular check and emergent action if any concerns are identified.

THE KNEE
Incidence
The incidence of vascular injury during total knee arthroplasty is slightly higher than during total hip arthroplasty[2–6] and has been reported between 0.057% and 0.19%.[2–6,31–34] Most injuries are thrombus formation secondary to indirect injury, commonly affecting the popliteal artery[2–6]; however, direct injury to vessels from a saw blade, the tip of a retractor, or overzealous posterior dissection may also occur. Vascular injury during revision surgery is more common with an incidence ranging from 0.19% to 0.36%.[2,4,5]

Risk Factors
Revision surgery remains the greatest risk factor for vascular injury, with an approximately 2 to 3 times increased risk compared with primary surgery.[2,4,5,32]

Matsen Ko and colleagues[32] carried out a US health care database study identifying 663 vascular injuries from 1,120,508 total knee arthroplasties. Along with revision surgery, they also identified peripheral vascular disease, weight loss, renal failure, coagulopathy, and metastatic cancer as risk factors.

DeLaurentis and colleagues[35] also identified underlying peripheral vascular disease as a risk factor for vascular injury. In their review of more than 1000 total knee arthroplasties, only 24 patients were identified with chronic lower limb ischemia; however, all 6 vascular injuries in their series occurred within this subgroup (25% incidence). Padegimas and colleagues[33] reported 4 of 13 vascular injuries had arterial calcification seen on preoperative radiographs.

African American race[4,33] and female gender[3,33] have also been suggested as risk factors for vascular injury.

Anatomy
The popliteal artery arises as a continuation of the superficial femoral artery as it passes through the adductor hiatus. It courses over the posterior capsule of the knee and branches into the anterior and posterior tibial arteries and peroneal artery as it passes beneath the soleal arch, on average 6 cm distal to the tibial articular surface.[36] It is tethered proximally at the adductor hiatus and distally at the soleal arch, as well as by its geniculate artery branches and (Fig. 4).

The popliteal artery gives rise to the 5 geniculate arteries: the superior medial, superior lateral, middle, inferior medial, and inferior lateral geniculate arteries. The superior lateral geniculate artery courses above the level of the lateral condyle of the femur, supplying the vastus lateralis muscle and anastomosing with the superior medial geniculate artery proximal to the patella. The superior lateral geniculate artery is at risk during lateral release for patellar tracking. The inferior lateral geniculate artery courses near the joint line proximal to the fibula head. It supplies the lateral meniscus, giving off prominent branches anterior to the popliteal hiatus and may cause bleeding from lateral meniscus resection.

In revision surgery, the popliteal artery may be more adherent to the posterior capsule within fibrous scar tissue, making it more susceptible to injury.

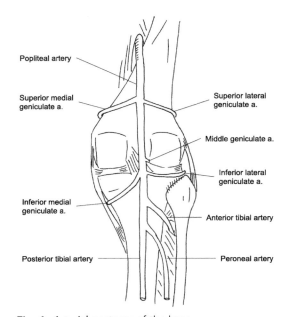

Fig. 4. Arterial anatomy of the knee.

Ninomiya and colleagues[37] performed a cadaver and MRI study reporting that the popliteal artery lies lateral to the posterior cruciate ligament (PCL) in 95% of knees. They found a retractor placed lateral to the PCL or greater than 1 cm into the posterior tissues placed the popliteal artery at risk. A retractor placed medial to the PCL was safe.

Yoo and colleagues[38] examined the location of the popliteal artery in extension and 90° flexion in young nonarthritic men. On the axial images, the popliteal artery was lateral to the PCL in 90%, an average of 3.9 mm from the capsule in extension, increasing to 7.6 mm at 90°. One centimeter distal to the joint (an approximation of the tibial cut level during total knee arthroplasty), the artery was 2.7 mm from the posterior cortex in extension, compared with 7.2 mm at 90°.

Farrington and colleagues[39] carried out a similar study; however, they used Doppler ultrasound in arthritic knees. The popliteal artery moved an average of 3.15 mm further from the posterior tibial cortex at 90° compared with extension; however, this increased safety margin only occurred in 61% of patients with previous total knee replacement.

The tibial and femoral cuts, along with any posterior dissection or debridement, should be carried out with the knee in flexion, to allow the greatest distance to the popliteal vessels.

Anatomic variation of the popliteal arterial tree may increase the risk of vascular injury. Tindall and colleagues[40] identified a 6% incidence of a "high origin anterior tibial artery." In these patients, the popliteal artery divides proximal to the popliteus, and the anterior tibial artery courses anterior to the popliteus in direct contact with the posterior tibia (Fig. 5). This highlights the potential danger of aberrant retractor placement or aggressive debridement around the posterolateral tibia. For this reason, the posterior retractor should not be placed deep, and in revision cases, a blunt-tipped retractor should be used because bone loss within the proximal tibia may bring the trifurcation closer to the tibial surface.

Mechanism of Injury

Vascular injuries during total knee arthroplasty are predominantly indirect injuries causing intimal tear and thrombotic occlusion.[2–6] Atheromatous vessels are more susceptible to mechanical pressure, which may lead to plaque fracture, causing embolization or thrombus and ischemia.[41–44] The popliteal artery is tethered proximally at the adductor hiatus and distally by the soleal arch, and the superficial femoral artery may be further tethered by a tourniquet above, making it susceptible to indirect mechanical injury during manipulation of the knee. Correction of a severe fixed flexion contracture may similarly cause indirect injury to the tethered and chronically shortened artery.

Less commonly, the popliteal artery may be directly lacerated by a saw blade, retractor tip, or other sharp instrument.[3,6,31,44,45] It has also been suggested that the sharp posterior edge

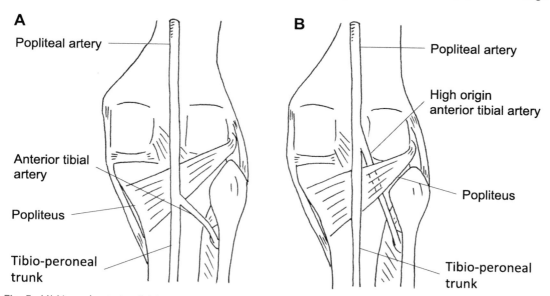

Fig. 5. (*A*) Normal anterior tibial artery origin. (*B*) High origin anterior tibial artery running anterior to popliteus, in contact with the posterior cortex of the tibia.

of the proximal tibia, after the proximal tibial resection, may cause direct injury if the knee is allowed to significantly hyperextend.[36]

Rarely, popliteal aneurysms may preexist and are susceptible to thrombosis during the low flow state induced by tourniquet use.[44]

As in the hip, a more subtle vascular injury may lead to pseudoaneurysm formation or arteriovenous fistula.[6,31,44–48] This has been reported related to popliteal artery injury, but may also arise from injury to the superior lateral geniculate artery during lateral release or by shear injury,[6,49,50] or the inferior lateral geniculate artery.[50,51] If performing a lateral release, an attempt should be made to identify and protect the superior lateral geniculate artery. When the tourniquet is released before closure, the lateral release should be carefully inspected for ongoing bleeding. Care can be taken to avoid injury to the inferior lateral geniculate artery by leaving a small rim of lateral meniscus anterior to the popliteal hiatus and cauterizing the vessel branches supplying the meniscus in this area.[51]

Patients with previous peripheral arterial bypass graft must be identified, as they are high risk of reocclusion during total knee arthroplasty. Turner and colleagues[52] identified 2 acute arterial occlusions among 10 patients with previous ipsilateral bypass grafts. Of note, 1 occlusion occurred among 7 patients in whom a tourniquet was used, and 1 occlusion occurred among 3 patients with tourniquetless surgery, demonstrating graft occlusion remains a risk with or without tourniquet use.

Preoperative Assessment

As per the hip, preoperative assessment for total knee arthroplasty should always include a thorough vascular history and examination.

In addition to the history and examination outlined for the preoperative assessment for total hip arthroplasty, the popliteal fossa should be palpated for a popliteal aneurysm. A Doppler ultrasound may be helpful in differentiating a popliteal aneurysm from a common Baker cyst. Radiographs of the knee should be examined for vascular calcification. If there are any concerns, then ABIs should be obtained.

A referral for vascular consultation and consideration of further imaging and potential intervention has been suggested in patients with significant risk identified on history and examination, an ABI less than 0.9, or vascular calcification seen on radiograph.[41,52]

The timing of vascular intervention is contentious, owing to the risk of bypass occlusion during total knee arthroplasty.[53,54] Calligaro and colleagues[54] suggested for patients with an ABI less than 0.5 that bypass surgery should not be performed before total knee arthroplasty because of the risk of intraoperative occlusion. They suggest a tourniquetless knee replacement after preoperative angiography, which allows for emergent revascularization if necessary. Nevertheless, in such cases, the authors consult with a vascular surgeon for a determination of order of intervention and whether there is sufficient circulation for a safe recovery from a knee replacement.

Tourniquet Use

The bloodless field achieved by tourniquet use may provide improved visualization, surgical ease, and a dry bone surface for improved cementing. This is balanced against a potential risk of neurologic or vascular injury, which may occur from direct tourniquet pressure causing intimal injury and thrombosis[55] or by tethering of the superficial femoral artery and increased risk of injury during manipulation of the knee.[56] Systemic risks of tourniquet use must also be considered.

In a recent meta-analysis, Ahmed and colleagues[57] found that tourniquet use in total knee arthroplasty led to increased serious adverse events (including deep vein thrombosis/pulmonary embolism, infection, nerve damage, reoperation, and mortality), increased pain scores, and marginally increased length of hospital stay. The only advantage of tourniquet use was decreased surgical time.

In patients with significant risk for vascular compromise, such as known peripheral vascular disease, absent pulses or vascular calcification on radiographs, tourniquetless surgery should be considered.[35,58] If a tourniquet is deemed necessary, a 5000 unit intravenous bolus of heparin can be administered before tourniquet inflation and reversed with protamine sulfate at the completion of the operation.[58]

If a tourniquet is used, the tourniquet size, type, and limb occlusion pressure should be optimized for each patient, and tourniquet time should be kept as short as practically possible. The tourniquet should be let down before closure to allow identification and control of bleeding. In high-risk situations, such as revision surgery, the tourniquet can be let down before liner insertion, allowing access to the back of the knee.

Presentation and Management

Vascular complications associated with total knee arthroplasty may present as acute intraoperative hemorrhage, postoperative ischemia, or false aneurysm.

Acute hemorrhage is usually identified at the time of surgery and mandates vascular surgery involvement for emergent repair. After identifying the vascular injury, proximal control can be achieved by direct pressure and tourniquet inflation until the vascular surgeon arrives. A sterile tourniquet can be applied if a tourniquet was not applied before draping the leg. Open repair is the treatment of choice in this situation, and depending on the degree of vessel injury, may be directly repaired, addressed with patch angioplasty, end-to-end anastomosis, interposition graft, or bypass.[5,41]

More commonly, vascular injury during total knee arthroplasty presents as acute ischemia.[2–6] The orthopedic surgeon should examine pedal pulses before and at the completion of every surgery, and if there is any suspicion of ischemia, an emergent vascular consultation and angiography should be sought.

In patients presenting with ischemia, endovascular techniques have become increasingly popular over traditional open techniques.[5] In their review of 49 vascular injuries, Troutman and colleagues[5] observed the transition from open to endovascular techniques, with only 6% of patients successfully treated with endovascular intervention before 2002, compared with 59% after 2002. The same investigators have cautioned against use of thrombectomy alone, being successful in only 28% of cases, with the remainder requiring a second procedure.[2] In another series,[54] they identified 10 patients treated with thrombectomy alone (6), sympathectomy alone (2), fasciotomy alone (1), and delayed bypass (1), which led to 7 amputations and 1 death. Because of these terrible outcomes, they recommended bypass surgery; however, with the increased utilization of endovascular interventions, they now recommend thrombectomy combined with assessment of the underlying vascular injury and commonly stenting.[5]

In any case of lower limb ischemia, fasciotomies must be considered, particularly with an ischemic time greater than 4 to 6 hours.[2]

False aneurysms are often diagnosed late[5,47,50] and may present as recurrent hemarthroses,[48,50] thrombosis/distal ischemia secondary to embolism,[48] or neurologic deficit secondary to mass effect.[59,60] Diagnosis may be difficult and may be delayed by days to many months.[5,47,50] A Doppler ultrasound can be useful in identifying false aneurysms in the patient with posterior pain and swelling. False aneurysms are readily amenable to endovascular management,[5] which may involve coil embolization, thrombin injection, or stent graft exclusion.[5,46]

Outcomes

The outcomes of vascular injury during total knee arthroplasty may be severe. Matsen Ko and colleagues[32] reported a 20-fold increase in mortality in patients with vascular injury. Outcomes are related to the timing of diagnosis and vascular intervention. Calligaro and colleagues[2] reported no deaths or loss of limb in 24 patients; however, 44% of patients presenting with acute ischemia were not diagnosed until greater than 24 hours postoperatively. Those patients with a delayed diagnosis had an increased rate of fasciotomies and foot drop. Abularrage and colleagues[4] had a 10% amputation rate among 20 patients, with the patients with amputation being diagnosed at day 12 and day 15.

Parvizi and colleagues[3] had 1 patient present at 12 days postoperatively who underwent an amputation. Among their remaining 10 patients, they reported 1 periprosthetic infection, 1 nerve palsy, 5 fasciotomies, and 1 skin graft. Bernhoff and colleagues[45] identified 32 patients with vascular injury, one of which required an amputation and 25 of 32 who had residual symptoms. Of the 7 patients with good outcomes, 6 were diagnosed and treated at the time of the index surgery.

With early diagnosis and treatment, these severe complications may potentially be avoided. Padegimas and colleagues[33] carried out early revascularization procedures on 12 patients diagnosed on the same day and 1 patient on day 1 post-surgery. All had good outcomes. Karanam and colleagues[34] treated 8 patients identified immediately postoperatively with endovascular intervention with good outcomes. One patient identified at day 3 went on to require an amputation.

Those with delayed revascularization often require fasciotomy. Vegari and colleagues[61] highlighted the very high complication rate in this group, reviewing 6 patients who required fasciotomy postvascular injury during total knee arthroplasty. All patients experienced a complication, including 1 amputation, 2 periprosthetic infections, 1 fasciitis, 1 cellulitis, 1 nonhealing wound, and 2 neurologic deficits. Early recognition and treatment of ischemia may reduce the need for fasciotomies and the associated complications.

SUMMARY

Vascular injuries during hip and knee arthroplasty are rare, but potentially life and limb threatening. Injuries may be reduced through careful preoperative assessment and planning, along with a knowledge of relevant vascular anatomy and careful surgical technique. Diagnosis, communication with the entire team, exposure and temporary control, and emergent vascular surgery consultation are the cornerstones of management for direct injuries. No surgery is complete without an immediate postoperative assessment of pedal pulses, allowing early recognition and intervention for ischemic injuries, which may lead to improved outcomes.

CLINICS CARE POINTS

Hip:

- Always carry out preoperative and postoperative vascular examinations.
- Consider a retroperitoneal approach for revision of a medialized acetabular component/intrapelvic cement removal.
- Careful placement of the anterior retractor over the superior portion of the anterior wall, between bone and capsule, helps avoid direct vascular injury.
- Place screws only in the safe quadrants: posterosuperior and posteroinferior.

Knee:

- Always carry out preoperative and postoperative vascular examinations.
- Consider tourniquetless surgery, particularly in high-risk patients.
- Careful placement of the posterior retractor on bone, medial to the posterior cruciate ligament, helps avoid vascular injury.

DISCLOSURE

M.W.J. Street has nothing to disclose. L.C. Howard is part of a division that accepts fellowship funding from industry and has no relevant disclosures to this topic. M.E. Neufeld is part of a division that accepts fellowship funding from industry and has no relevant disclosures to this topic. B.A. Masri is Deputy Editor for *Joint Reconstruction, Journal of Bone and Joint Surgery*. Dr Masri is a consultant for Stryker and the institution receives support from Stryker, Smith and Nephew and Zimmer.

REFERENCES

1. Nachbur B, Meyer RP, Verkkala K, et al. The mechanisms of severe arterial injury in surgery of the hip joint. Clin Orthop Relat Res 1979;141:122–33.
2. Calligaro KD, Dougherty MJ, Ryan S, et al. Acute arterial complications associated with total hip and knee arthroplasty. J Vasc Surg 2003;38(6):1170–5.
3. Parvizi J, Pulido L, Slenker N, et al. Vascular injuries after total joint arthroplasty. J Arthroplasty 2008;23(8):1115–21.
4. Abularrage CJ, Weiswasser JM, DeZee KJ, et al. Predictors of lower extremity arterial injury after total knee or total hip arthroplasty. J Vasc Surg 2008;47(4):803–7.
5. Troutman DA, Dougherty MJ, Spivack AI, et al. Updated strategies to treat acute arterial complications associated with total knee and hip arthroplasty. J Vasc Surg 2013;58(4):1037–42.
6. Avisar E, Haward Elvey M, Bar-Ziv Y, et al. Severe vascular complications and intervention following elective total hip and knee replacement: a 16-year retrospective analysis. J Orthop 2015;12:151–5.
7. Shoenfeld NA, Stuchin SA, Pearl R, et al. The management of vascular injuries associated with total hip arthroplasty. J Vasc Surg 1990;11(4):549–55.
8. Lazarides MK, Arvanitis DP, Dayantas JN. Iatrogenic arterial trauma associated with hip joint surgery: an overview. Eur J Vasc Surg 1991;5:549–56.
9. Bergqvist D, Carlsson AS, Ericsson BF. Vascular complications after total hip arthroplasty. Acta Orhop Scand 1983;54:157–63.
10. Alshameeri Z, Bajekal R, Varty K, et al. Iatrogenic vascular injuries during arthroplasty of the hip. Bone Joint J 2015;97-B:1447–55.
11. Fukunishi S, Okahisa S, Fukui T, et al. Significance of preoperative 3D-CT angiography for localization of the femoral artery in complicated THA. J Orthop Sci 2014;19:457–64.
12. Reiley MA, Bond D, Branick RI, et al. Vascular complications following total hip arthroplasty: a review of the literature and a report of two cases. Clin Orthop Relat Res 1984;186:23–8.
13. Grigoris P, Roberts P, McMinn DJW, et al. A technique for removing an intrapelvic acetabular cup. J Bone Joint Surg Br 1993;75-B:25–7.
14. Asemota D, Passano B, Feng JE, et al. Preoperative optimization for vascular involvement complicating revision total hip arthroplasty. Arthrop Today 2018;4:411–6.
15. Wera GD, Ting NT, Della Valle CJ, et al. External iliac artery injury complicating prosthetic hip resection for infection. J Arthroplasty 2009;25(4):660.e1-4.
16. Kawasaki Y, Egawa H, Hamada D, et al. Location of intrapelvic vessels around the acetabulum assessed by three-dimensional computed tomographic angiography: prevention of vascular-related complications in total hip arthroplasty. J Orthop Sci 2012;17:397–406.
17. Feugier P, Fessy MH, Bejui J, et al. Acetabular anatomy and the relationship with pelvic vascular

structures: implications in hip surgery. Surg Radiol Anat 1997;19:85–90.

18. Kirkpatrick JS, Callaghan JJ, Vandemark RM, et al. The relationship of the intrapelvic vasculature to the acetabulum. Implications in screw-fixation acetabular components. Clin Orthop Relat Res 1990;258:183–90.

19. Rue JH, Inoue N, Mont MA. Current overview of neurovascular structures in hip arthroplasty: anatomy, preoperative evaluation, approaches, and operative techniques to avoid complications. Orthopaedics 2004;27(1):73–81.

20. Wasielewski RC, Cooperstein LA, Kruger MP, et al. Acetabular anatomy and the transacetabular fixation of screws in total hip arthroplasty. J Bone Joint Surg Am 1990;72:501–8.

21. Meldrum R, Lance Johansen R. Safe screw placement in acetabular revision surgery. J Arthroplasty 2001;16(8):953–60.

22. Keating EM, Ritter MA, Faris PM. Structures at risk from medially placed acetabular screws. J Bone Joint Surg Am 1990;72:509–11.

23. Hwang SK. Vascular injury during total hip arthroplasty: the anatomy of the acetabulum. Int Orthop 1994;18:29–31.

24. Chan SW, Wong HC, Wong KY. Lower limb ischaemia complicating total hip arthroplasty. J Orthop Trauma Rehab 2012;16:29–32.

25. Shubert D, Madoff S, Milillo R, et al. Neurovascular structure proximity to acetabular retractors in total hip arthroplasty. J Arthroplasty 2015;30:145–8.

26. Girard J, Blairon A, Wavreille G, et al. Total hip arthroplasty revision in case of intra-pelvic cup migration: describing a surgical strategy. Orthop Traumatol-Surg Res 2011;97:191–200.

27. Maeckelberg L, Simon J, Naudie D, et al. Removal of an intra-pelvic socket: description of a safe surgical algorithm. Acta Orthop Belg 2012;78:152–8.

28. Bach CM, Steingruber I, Wimmer C, et al. False aneurysm 14 years after total hip arthroplasty. J Arthroplasty 2000;15:535–8.

29. An S, Shen H, Feng M, et al. Femoral artery injury during total hip arthroplasty. Arthrop Today 2018; 4:459–63.

30. Mavrogenis AF, Rossi G, Rimondi E, et al. Embolisation for vascular injuries complicating elective orthopaedic surgery. Eur J Vasc Endovasc Surg 2011; 42:676–83.

31. Pal A, Clarke JMF, Cameron AEP. Case series and literature review: popliteal artery injury following total knee replacement. Int J Surg 2010;8:430–5.

32. Matsen Ko LJ, DeHart ML, Yoo JU, et al. Popliteal artery injury associated with total knee arthroplasty: trends, costs and risk factors. J Arthroplasty 2014; 29:1181–4.

33. Padegimas EM, Levicoff EA, McGinley AD, et al. Vascular complications after total knee arthroplasty

– a single institution experience. J Arthroplasty 2016;31:1583–8.

34. Karanam LSP, Busireddy NR, Baddam SR, et al. Acute thrombotic occlusion after total knee arthroplasty: role of endovascular management. J Clin Orthop Trauma 2018;9:121–4.

35. DeLaurentis DA, Levistsky KA, Booth RE, et al. Arterial and ischaemic aspects of total knee arthroplasty. Am J Surg 1992;164:237–40.

36. Kim D, Orron DE, Skillman JJ. Surgical significance of popliteal arterial variants. A unified angiographic classification. Ann Surg 1989;210:776–81.

37. Ninomiya JT, Dean JC, Goldberg VM. Injury to the popliteal artery and its anatomic location in total knee arthroplasty. J Arthroplasty 1999;14(7):803–9.

38. Yoo JH, Chang CB. The location of the popliteal artery in extension and 90 degree knee flexion measured on MRI. Knee 2009;16(2):143–8.

39. Farrington WJ, Charnley GJ, Harries SR, et al. The position of the popliteal artery in the arthritic knee. J Arthroplasty 1999;14(7):800–2.

40. Tindall AJ, Shetty AA, James KD, et al. Prevalence and surgical significance of a high-origin anterior tibial artery. J Orthop Surg 2006;14(1):13–6.

41. Butt U, Samuel R, Sahu A, et al. Arterial injury in total knee arthroplasty. J Arthroplasty 2010;25(8):1311–8.

42. Rand JA. Vascular complications after total knee arthroplasty. Report of three cases. J Arthroplasty 1987;2(2):89–93.

43. Kumar SN, Chapman JA, Rawlins I. Vascular injuries in total knee arthroplasty. A review of the problem with special reference to the possible effects of the tourniquet. J Arthroplasty 1998;13(2):211–6.

44. Holmberg A, Milbrink J, Bergqvist D. Arterial complications after knee arthroplasty: 4 cases and review of the literature. Acta Orthop Scand 1996;67(1):75–8.

45. Bernhoff K, Rudstrom H, Gedeborg R, et al. Popliteal artery injury during knee replacement. A population-based nationwide study. Bone Joint J 2013;95-B:1645–9.

46. Geertsema D, Defoort KC, van Hellemondt GG. Popliteal pseudoaneurysm after total knee arthroplasty. A report of 3 cases. J Arthroplasty 2012; 27(8):1581.e1-4.

47. Hozack WJ, Cole PA, Gardner R, et al. Popliteal aneurysm after total knee arthroplasty. Case reports and review of the literature. J Arthroplasty 1990;5(4):301–5.

48. Ibrahim M, Booth RE, Clark TW. Embolization of traumatic pseudoaneurysms after total knee arthroplasty. J Arthroplasty 2004;19(1):123–8.

49. Saini P, Meena S, Malhotra R, et al. Pseudoaneurysm of the superior lateral genicular artery: case report of a rare complication after total knee arthroplasty. Patient Saf Surg 2013;7:15.

50. Katsimihas M, Robinson D, Thornton M, et al. Therapeutic embolization of the geniculate arteries for

recurrent haemarthrosis after total knee arthroplasty. J Arthroplasty 2001;16(7):935–7.

51. Pai VS. Traumatic aneurysm of the inferior lateral geniculate artery after total knee replacement. J Arthroplasty 1999;14(5):633–4.

52. Turner NS, Pagnano MW, Sim FH. Total knee arthroplasty after ipsilateral peripheral arterial bypass graft. Acute arterial occlusion is a risk with or without tourniquet use. J Arthroplasty 2001; 16(3):317–21.

53. Garabekyan T, Oliashirazi A, Winters K. The value of immediate preoperative vascular examination in an at-risk patient for total knee arthroplasty. Orthopaedics 2011;34(1):52.

54. Calligaro KD, DeLaurentis DA, Booth RE, et al. Acute arterial thrombosis associated with total knee arthroplasty. J Vasc Surg 1994;20(6):927–32.

55. Parfenchuck T, Young T. Intraoperative arterial occlusion in total knee joint arthroplasty. J Arthroplasty 1994;9(2):217–20.

56. McAuley CE, Steed DL, Webster MW. Arterial complications of total knee replacement. Arch Surg 1984;119(8):960–2.

57. Ahmed I, Chawla A, Underwood M, et al. Time to reconsider the routine use of tourniquets in total knee arthroplasty surgery. Bone Joint J 2021;103-B(5):830–9.

58. Smith DE, McGraw RW, Taylor DC, et al. Arterial complications and total knee arthroplasty. J Am Acad Orthop Surg 2001;9(4):253–7.

59. Sandoval E, Ortega FJ, Garcia-Rayo MR, et al. Popliteal pseudoaneurysm after total knee arthroplasty secondary to intraoperative arterial injury with a surgical pin. J Arthroplasty 2008;23(8):1239.e7-11.

60. O'Connor JV, Stocks G, Crabtree JD, et al. Popliteal pseudoaneurysm following total knee arthroplasty. J Arthroplasty 1998;13(7):830–2.

61. Vegari DN, Rangavajjula AV, Dilorio TM, et al. Fasciotomy following total knee arthroplasty: beware of terrible outcome. J Arthroplasty 2014;29:355–9.

Sepsis and Total Joint Arthroplasty

Karan M. Patel, BA[a], Simon C. Mears, MD, PhD[b], Charles Lowry Barnes, MD[b],
Jeffrey B. Stambough, MD[b], Benjamin M. Stronach, MS, MD[b],*

KEYWORDS

- Sepsis • Periprosthetic joint infection (PJI) • SIRS criteria • Total joint arthroplasty (TJA)
- Quick Sequential Organ Failure Assessment score (qSOFA) score • Bacteremia • Severe sepsis
- Sepsis treatment

KEY POINTS

- Periprosthetic joint infection (PJI) following a total joint arthroplasty (TJA) is a difficult problem to diagnose and treat. If left untreated, the infection can progress to sepsis leading to life-threatening consequences.
- The definition of sepsis is still debated, and this makes diagnosis and treatment problematic for physicians. Both SIRS criteria and qSOFA score have their own strengths and weaknesses.
- Sepsis that occurs in patients who have undergone TJA can occur due to PJI or independently without PJI. There are not clear guidelines to follow when treating these patients, but case reports have examined the severity of sepsis in patients who have undergone TJA.
- Urgent diagnosis and treatment of sepsis is important to improve outcomes; this may necessitate giving antibiotics before joint fluid can be obtained, especially in the setting of bacteremia.
- Sepsis may occur during the perioperative period while treating a prosthetic joint infection, and the surgeon should monitor the patient closely because this often necessitates intensive care admission.

INTRODUCTION

Periprosthetic joint infection (PJI) is a difficult complication to treat and is a common cause for revision total joint arthroplasty (TJA).[1] PJI is defined as an infection involving the prosthesis and surrounding soft tissue and bone and can occur acutely after the index procedure or in a delayed fashion. Acute infection is typically attributed to an intraoperative source or can occur due to wound breakdown or bacterial seeding of a postoperative hematoma. In contrast, delayed infection can occur at any given time throughout the patient's life after joint replacement. In the setting of delayed infection, the infectious source is typically hematogenous in nature. The patient typically develops an infection in a site remote to the joint, such as pneumonia or an abscess, and bacteria then enters the blood stream and seeds the joint. This is a difficult problem to prevent because the human joint has a limited immune response in an avascular environment coupled with the presence of an artificial surface that the body is unable to actively protect.

Sepsis is a medical emergency resulting from microorganisms infiltrating the body, which are then spread through the vascular system; this leads to a physiologic response that can result in organ damage, shock, and death. Although the definition and clinical diagnostic criteria of sepsis have evolved within the past 3 decades,

[a] University of Arkansas for Medical Sciences, 4301 West Markham Street, Slot 531, Little Rock, AR 72205, USA;
[b] Department of Orthopedic Surgery, University of Arkansas for Medical Sciences, 4301 West Markham Street, Slot 531, Little Rock, AR 72205, USA
* Corresponding author.
E-mail address: BStronach@uams.edu

Orthop Clin N Am 53 (2022) 13–24
https://doi.org/10.1016/j.ocl.2021.08.008
0030-5898/22/© 2021 Elsevier Inc. All rights reserved.

many physicians rely on specific diagnostic findings comprising the systemic inflammatory response syndrome (SIRS) criteria to include fever, tachycardia, tachypnea, and leukocytosis[2] (Table 1). An individual must exhibit 2 or more of the SIRS criteria that stem from an infection to formally be diagnosed with sepsis.[2]

Sepsis is a rare complication in patients who have undergone a TJA. Sepsis can develop in the immediate postoperative setting, or in a remote time frame unrelated to the index arthroplasty procedure. Sepsis is a potentially fatal disease process; therefore, timely treatment is critical to save lives. We provide a review on the diagnosis and treatment of sepsis in patients who have undergone TJA, both with and without concurrent PJI. There is limited literature available on the topic of sepsis in the setting of TJA to guide treatment, so we provide general content on both topics to help better inform the reader. We also review the literature that is available on this specific topic, which is primarily limited to case series and case reports.

Total Joint Arthroplasty and Prosthetic Joint Infection

It has recently been estimated that 1.5 million total hip arthroplasties (THA) and total knee arthroplasties (TKA) are performed annually in the United States.[3] This number is expected to grow to more than 4 million annual TJA procedures by the year 2030.[4] Approximately 2% of patients who have undergone a TJA develop PJI.[5] Infection accounts for 14.8% of THA revisions and has been reported to be the cause for up to 25.2% of TKA revisions.[6] As the number of TJA increases, we will assuredly see a corresponding increase in the number of PJIs in the future.

The clinical presentation of PJI varies drastically and depends on numerous factors including the causative microorganisms, host, immune response, and the joint involved. Common signs of PJI can include joint pain, swelling, and drainage. PJI has had many definitions throughout the years given the broad spectrum of associated symptoms. This situation has led the Musculoskeletal Infection Society to propose universal criteria for the diagnosis of PJI (Table 2).[7] PJI is diagnosed when at least one major criterion is met, or the patient has an additive score of greater than 6 based on minor criteria.

Periprosthetic joint infection treatment

Chronic PJI is typically treated with a 2-stage exchange arthroplasty in the United States[8] as opposed to Europe where 1-stage exchange arthroplasty is often the preferred treatment. In a 2-stage treatment course, the first stage begins with the removal of the infected prosthesis along with excision of all involved soft tissue and bone. Multiple soft tissue cultures (a minimum of 3 samples has been proposed) should then be collected to identify the microorganism responsible for the infection.[8] A static or articulating cement spacer infused with antibiotics is then placed within the joint.

Static spacers do not allow for joint range of motion and are typically not made to allow full weight-bearing. An articulating spacer provides maintenance of joint motion and partial or full weight-bearing depending on the construct. Articulating spacers have shown comparable efficacy with static spacers in terms of infection eradication and offer the potential advantage of preserved joint range of motion during the treatment course with simplification of the second-stage reconstruction.[9]

Broad-spectrum antibiotics are typically administered initially in the immediate postoperative setting as the surgeon awaits culture results if the organism is not known before surgery. An infectious disease specialist should help direct antibiotic selection and monitoring.

Table 1	
Symptoms/lab values and diagnostic score required for both systemic inflammatory response syndrome criteria and Quick Sequential Organ Failure Assessment score in the diagnosis of sepsis '	
SIRS Criteria (≥2)	**qSOFA Score (≥2)**
Temperature > 38 or < 36°C c	Systolic blood pressure < 100 mm Hg
Respiratory rate > 22/min	Respiratory rate > 20/min
Heart rate > 90 bpm	Glasgow coma score ≤ 14
White blood cell count > 12,000 or < 4000	

Abbreviation: qSOFA, Quick Sequential Organ Failure Assessment.
   Data from International Clinical Pathology Journal and Federal Practioner: for the health care workers of the VA, DoD, and PHS.

Table 2
Expanded list of systemic inflammatory response syndrome criteria created in the second sepsis conference

Symptoms/Laboratory Test Results	Values
Hypotension	Systolic blood pressure < 100 mm Hg
High bilirubin	>4 mg/dL
Lactate	> 1 mmol/L
Platelet count	< 100,000 mcL
White blood cell count	> 12,000/mm^3 or < 4000/mm^3
Mottled skin	
Absent bowel sounds from ileus	
Reduced capillary refill of nail beds or skin	
aPTT	> 60 s or INR >5
Fever	> 38.3° C
Hypothermia	<36° C
Tachycardia	> 90 beat/min
Tachypnea	> 20 breaths/min
Creatinine	> 0.5 mg/dL
Altered mental status	
Reduced urine output	
Edema	
Arterial hypoxemia	<300 Pao$_2$/Fio$_2$
Hyperglycemia	> 140 mg/dL
Elevated procalcitonin levels in scrum	
Elevated c-reactive protein	

Abbreviations: aPTT, activated partial thromboplastin time; INR, international normalized ratio.
Data from Data from International Clinical Pathology Journal.

A more focused antibiotic can then be selected if the operative cultures identify an organisms.[8]

Stage 2 of the exchange arthroplasty involves the removal of the spacer and the placement of a new implant.[8] Significant variation remains in the timing for the second-stage procedure along with how best to determine if there is residual infection and whether antibiotics should be continued or stopped. A 3-month course of continued oral antibiotics after the second-stage reimplantation has shown benefit in preventing infection recurrence.[10]

Sepsis and Systemic Inflammatory Response Syndrome

Sepsis is a medical emergency resulting from an infectious agent infiltrating the body and spreading through the vascular system. The physiologic response to this is fever/hypothermia, tachycardia, tachypnea, and leukocytosis/leukopenia[11] (see Table 1). These symptoms can result in organ damage, septic shock, and death. There are approximately 300 cases of sepsis per 100,000 people in the United States annually[12] with a resultant $20 billion associated cost to the health care system.[13] Patients who develop sepsis are at greater risk for subsequent septic episodes and have 3.2 infections per patient-year compared with only 0.6 infections per patient-year in the control population.[14]

Pathophysiology of sepsis

Inflammation from sepsis is mediated by neutrophils and macrophages releasing cytokines such as tumor necrosis factor-alpha, interleukins, and prostaglandins.[11] The release of cytokines triggers consumption of anticoagulants in the body with a resultant inhibition of fibrinolysis and upregulation of the extrinsic coagulation cascade[11]; this can lead to end-organ damage and even disseminated intravascular coagulation, which is a life-threatening condition that is difficult to treat.

Viruses, bacteria, fungi, and parasites are all insulting agents known to cause sepsis. *Escherichia coli, Streptococcus pneumonia,* and *Staphylococcus aureus* are the most common causative bacterial microorganisms for sepsis and may or may not track to the bloodstream (ie, bacteremia).[15] Successful treatment of sepsis depends early diagnosis and immediate treatment with broad-spectrum antibiotics and intravenous (IV) fluids.[15]

History of the evolving definition of sepsis

The first formal definition of sepsis (termed sepsis 1) was proposed in 1992 when The Society of Critical Care Medicine (SCCM) and the American College of Chest Physicians (ACCP) held a combined conference to address the lack of consensus in the medical community on this topic.[2] This conference introduced and defined the concept of SIRS (see Table 1), which was defined as an exaggerated response of the body because of numerous potential stressors, including infection, trauma, surgery, and ischemia. SIRS was intended to be a tool for clinicians to more easily diagnose patients who would potentially develop sepsis for rapid initiation of treatment with fluids and broad-spectrum antibiotics.[16] The committee went on to define sepsis as the development of SIRS in the setting of infection.[2] The terms severe sepsis, which is "sepsis associated with organ dysfunction, hypoperfusion, or hypotension,[2]" and septic shock, which is "sepsis-induced hypotension persisting despite adequate fluid resuscitation,[2]" were also defined at this time.

The secondary goal of developing SIRS criteria was to provide standardization for the purposes of research regarding sepsis. SIRS criteria allowed clinicians to quickly and efficiently diagnose inflammatory diseases with the tools at their immediate disposal. More sophisticated tools may allow for improved specificity but were either not readily available or required excessive time to result, which is not clinically helpful because timing of diagnosis in the setting of sepsis is critical. Although SIRS was developed to help clinicians in the diagnoses of sepsis, there is a commonality of the SIRS criteria with numerous diseases with a resultant low specificity for sepsis based on positive SIRS criteria. Pancreatitis, trauma, and ischemia are a few of the many disease processes that can lead to positive SIRS criteria.[16]

Sepsis 1 was problematic for a variety of reasons. The definition and diagnostic criteria it proposed could not accurately predict sepsis. The major issue with SIRS criteria was that the symptoms were not specific to sepsis alone; sepsis was SIRS stemming from an infection[16]; this caused aseptic patients to be treated with septic therapies. Jones and Lowes[17] found that 95% of patients with bacteremia fulfilled SIRS criteria, but the positive predictive value of SIRS for bacteremia was only 7%. The lack of specificity of the SIRS criteria has been a problem in using SIRS to diagnose sepsis and has caused the definition of sepsis to evolve through the past several decades.

In 2001 the SCCM, ACCP, the European Society of Intensive Care Medicine, the American Thoracic Society, and the Surgical Infection Society met to update sepsis criteria based on the limitations of sepsis 1. Sepsis-2 expanded SIRS to 21 diagnostic criteria (see Table 2) when diagnosing or screening for sepsis. The term sepsis was retained and unaltered. The term severe sepsis was retained but slightly altered to sepsis complicated by organ dysfunction.[18] This conference also introduced the acronym Predisposition, Infection, Response, and Organ Dysfunction (PIRO) to better describe a septic episode (Table 3). The similar characteristics of the old and new definitions along with the expansion of SIRS criteria caused confusion and lack of standardization among physicians and researchers.[18] Critics took exception with the Sepsis-2 definition because it did not make any notable changes to the qualifying sepsis criteria and is still prone to overdiagnosis of sepsis.[18]

Sepsis-3, introduced in 2016, has not been universally accepted or adopted. The new definition of sepsis is "life threatening organ dysfunction due to a dysregulated host response to infection."[2] At this consensus meeting, experts recommended that physicians not use the SIRS criteria because of lack of specificity with regard to infection because positive SIRS criteria can occur due to trauma, burns, and pancreatitis (see Table 3).[18] SIRS criteria were replaced by the Quick Sequential Organ Failure Assessment (qSOFA, see Table 1). The qSOFA consists of 3 diagnostic criteria to screen for patients who could potentially develop sepsis including a systolic blood pressure less than 100 mm Hg, respiratory rate greater than 20 bpm, and a Glasgow coma score of 14 or less (qSOFA). A score of 2 or more is considered positive indicating increased

Table 3 Key findings from each conference held to define/redefine sepsis ·	
SEPSIS CONFERENCE 1 (1992)	• Four stages of sepsis were defined and established 1. SIRS Criteria exhibiting at least 2/4 symptoms (see Table 3). 2. Sepsis - host's systemic inflammatory response syndrome (SIRS) to an infection. 3. Severe sepsis - sepsis accompanied by organ dysfunction, hypoperfusion, or hypotension. 4. Septic shock - hypotension from sepsis untreatable even with adequate fluid intake.
SEPSIS CONFERENCE 2 (2001)	• The terms sepsis and severe sepsis were retained. • Others were omitted. SIRS Criteria was expanded to 21 symptoms/laboratory exams (see Table 4). • The acronym PIRO was introduced to better describe the sepsis episode. 1. Predisposition - represents all predisposing factors prior to the occurrence of sepsis. 2. Infection - includes the description of the infection (localization, sensitivity, virulence, etc.). 3. Response - is based on the acute reaction of the host mainly the inflammatory response. 4. Organ Dysfunction - is defined as the number of organs/organ systems affected and the gravity of the dysfunction.
SEPSIS CONFERENCE 3 (2016)	• New sepsis definition - "life threatening organ dysfunction due to a dysregulated host response to infection".[2] • SIRS criteria are no longer used to define sepsis. • Stage 1 - Severe sepsis - "is a life-threatening organ dysfunction due to a dysregulated host response to infection." • Stage 2 - Septic shock - this is a subset of sepsis where circulatory, cellular, and metabolic abnormalities are linked to an increase risk of mortality. • The sequential organ failure assessment (SOFA) score and quickSOFA (qSOFA) score were introduced which are based on multiple organ systems and replace SIRS criteria (see Table 3).

Data from International Clinical Pathology Journal and *Federal Practioner: for the health care workers of the VA, DoD, and PHS.*

risk of sepsis in patients with clinically suspected sepsis.[19] qSOFA was developed as a subset of the original SOFA score to provide a quicker and more practical tool to use in the emergency department for rapid sepsis screening. The full SOFA score analyzes the dysfunction of 5 organ systems (respiratory, cardiovascular, coagulation, renal, neurologic).[18] qSOFA was not intended to be diagnostic for sepsis, but as a warning for potential sepsis or rapid deterioration in patients with a suspected infection.[18]

Systemic inflammatory response syndrome criteria versus quick sequential organ failure assessment
The most drastic change in the evolution of the scoring system to clinically define sepsis (see Table 3) came in 2016 when the qSOFA score

replaced SIRS criteria. One reason for this change in Sepsis-3 was the difficulty of differentiating between inflammation from infectious (sepsis) and noninfectious sources.[20] Use of the SIRS criteria has led to potential overdiagnosis and unnecessary treatment of patients.[21] However, it is thought that overtreating patients who meet SIRS criteria but may not be septic is a safer alternative than potentially missing the diagnosis of a patient with sepsis. This remains a topic of controversy.[22]

Minderhoud and colleagues[23] studied antibiotic use in patients presenting to the emergency department (ED) with suspected sepsis in a cohort of 269 patients. All patients who exhibited 2 or more SIRS criteria were given antibiotics. The study found that 71% of the patients' symptoms were likely caused by a bacterial infection. Within the bacterial infection group, 58% met sepsis criteria (2008 definition), 30% met severe sepsis criteria, 9.5% had hypotension due to sepsis, and 3% suffered septic shock.[23] Many of the patients in this study would not have fit the sepsis-3 definition even though they received antibiotic treatment.

Dykes and colleagues[19] conducted a retrospective study to compare the effectiveness of SIRS to qSOFA in identifying sepsis. The study population was composed of 481veterans admitted to the intensive care unit (ICU) with a suspicion of early sepsis treated with empirical antibiotics. The study found that the qSOFA score was not a suitable replacement for SIRS criteria. The qSOFA score was found to have a higher specificity but lower sensitivity than SIRS criteria. This resulted in cases of sepsis going undetected in the qSOFA group. The increased specificity of qSOFA helps to decrease the potential for the inclusion of patients due to false-positive results, whereas the low sensitivity means it may be a poor screening tool. However, the lack of specificity with SIRS can lead to unneeded antibiotic administration, which carries the risk for harm to the patient and increased cost of care. In practice, both the qSOFA score and SIRS criteria are useful in the diagnosis of sepsis depending on the presentation of the patient and how these tools are applied clinically.

Sepsis in the emergency department

Sepsis is common in the emergency department and can lead to CU admission. Acute triage and early recognition are key in delivering quality care. The Surviving Sepsis Campaign, a global organization founded to lower sepsis mortality rates by bringing professional groups together, does not currently endorse any single screening tool for the identification of sepsis because of the aforementioned reasons. Recent studies have found that the National Early Warning Score (NEWS) has greater sensitivity to both qSOFA scores and SIRS criteria[24] in the setting of the ED (Table 4). Sepsis should be considered in any patient with a score greater than 5 in the setting of known infection in the NEWS system. In the ED, NEWS had increased sensitivity when compared with SIRS and qSOFA but lacked in specificity.[25] This observation supports the use of NEWS as a screening tool in this setting instead of the SIRS or qSOFA scoring systems.

Patients with suspected sepsis are administered fluids and broad-spectrum antibiotic medication, along with numerous other appropriate therapies, as the physician works to identify the

Table 4 National early warning score (NEWS)						
Physiologic	**3**	**2 1**	**0**	**1**	**2**	**3**
Parameters						
Respiration Rate (BPM)	≤8	9–11	12–20		21–24	≥25
Oxygen Saturation (%)	≤91	92–93 94–95	>96			
Any Supplemental Oxygen		yes	no			
Temperature (degrees C)	≤35.0	35.1–36.0	36.1–38.0	38.1–39.0	≥39.1	
Systolic Blood Pressure (mm Hg)	≤90	91–100	101–110	111–219		≥220
Level of Consciousness			Awake			Verbal, Pain, Unresponsive
Heart Rate (beats/min)	≤40	41–50	51–90	91–110	111–130	≥ 131

Data from Open Access Emergency Medicine.

source of the patient's illness.[15,24] The first priority in the treatment of sepsis is resuscitation of the patient with fluids because the pathophysiology of sepsis causes the loss of intravascular fluids from vascular leakage.[24] Timing of fluid administration is imperative because the mortality rate is lower in patients who receive fluids within 30 minutes of diagnosis.[26] The second priority is optimizing the fluid volume of resuscitation, which has been shown to reduce mortality rates.[26] The ideal fluid volume is determined by multiple physiologic factors with a goal to get the mean arterial pressure to 65 mm Hg or greater. The ideal fluid for resuscitation is unclear in the literature, but balanced crystalloids seem to be superior to normal saline[27] in patients with sepsis. Antibiotics selection and timing are also critical in lowering mortality rates. Broad-spectrum antibiotics should be administered within an hour of diagnosis. The change from broad-spectrum antibiotics to targeted therapy should occur swiftly if and when the specific organisms is identified.[21]

A procedure may be required to aid in the treatment, and elimination, of the infectious source from the patient. This procedure depends on the type and location of infection within the body and can include a wide spectrum of options from lancing of abscesses or placement of a drain up to an open surgical debridement of the infected area. The Surviving Sepsis Campaign guidelines recommend decompression and drainage within 12 hours of diagnosis. Open surgery is typically indicated as a last resort, and the risk of surgery and overall stability of the patient must be weighed against the potential benefit the surgery could provide. Surgery carries the risk of accelerated death and further damage from the procedure and associated anesthesia if the patient is not adequately stabilized.[28]

If the patient does not quickly improve after administering fluids and broad-spectrum antibiotics, it is recommended that further monitoring of the patient be undertaken to include urine output, blood gases, lactate, hemoglobin, and glucose. The physician should have a low threshold for transfer to the ICU if the patient does not rapidly stabilize with the initiation of treatment.[28]

Once sepsis is diagnosed in the emergency room in a patient with PJI, timely administration of broad-spectrum antibiotics is important. A 1-hour window[29] is recommended to improve mortality because the focus is on life-saving treatment, but this gives little time for aspiration of the infected joint; this may mean that the aspiration of the infected joint must occur after giving broad-spectrum IV antibiotics, which can decrease the likelihood of identifying the offending organism from joint culture.[30] Culture-negative PJI is less likely to be successfully treated because empirical therapy, instead of focused therapy, is provided.[31] There may be a chance to quickly aspirate a knee, whereas the hip joint usually requires either fluoroscopic or ultrasound guidance and it is unlikely this can be accomplished within the hour of opportunity.

Sepsis in Patients Undergoing Total Joint Arthroplasty

Incidence and causes

The incidence of surgically acquired sepsis has decreased 10-fold in the field of hip arthroplasty because advances in surgical procedures, sterile technique, and prophylactic bacterial treatment. The current rate of sepsis among primary THA patients is 0.5% or less. Most cases now are not due to surgical contamination, but foreign bacteria from other parts of the body with an overall 1% infection rate of THA over the life of the implant.[32] Patient education about early warning signs of an infection is an important process to lower the risk for developing sepsis.

Bohl and colleagues[33] examined the incidence and sources of sepsis following TJA. The study identified 117,935 (45,612 THA, 72,323 TKA) patients aged 18 to 80 year old who had undergone TJA from the years 2005 to 2013. Only 402 (0.34%) patients developed sepsis beyond the 30-day postoperative period after joint replacement. Sepsis from urinary tract infection (UTI) accounted for 124 (31%) cases. SSI was responsible for 110 (27%) cases, and pneumonia accounted for 60 (15%) cases. Twenty-one patients (5%) had infections that came from multiple sources, and 129 (32%) cases of sepsis were from an unidentifiable source[33] (Fig. 1). The findings from this study can be useful as a step-by-step guide for the clinical workup for suspected sepsis following TJA to include evaluation of the surgical site along with workup for UTI and pneumonia.

Bacteremia

Bacteremia is defined as the presence of bacteria within an individual's bloodstream, but as used in the literature it is an infection of the blood that leads to a disease process. The terms bacteremia and sepsis are distinct terms, although they are interchangeably used in the literature. Sepsis is the clinical condition that involves inflammation with other symptoms stemming from an infection. Sepsis with bacteremia

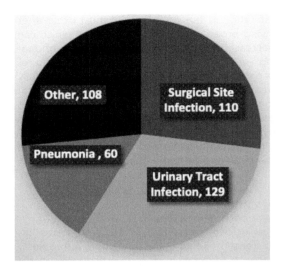

Fig. 1. Causes of sepsis in the 402 of 117,935 patients who have undergone total hip arthroplasty or total knee arthroplasty.[41] (*Data from* the Journal of arthroplasty.)

or sepsis stemming from bacteremia is also known as blood culture-positive sepsis. Blood culture-negative sepsis is a case of sepsis in whoch the culture does not have resultant growth. The confusion of terminology in the literature makes the disease process difficult to study and effectively communicate.

It has been approximated that pathogens are not isolated in 30% to 50%[34] of suspected sepsis cases. The patient then requires treatment with broad-spectrum antimicrobials as opposed to targeted therapy. Studies have found that patients with culture-positive sepsis have higher mortality rates than their culture-negative counterparts and are also more likely to exhibit multiple organ system complications.[34] Culture-negative sepsis sounds counterintuitive given that sepsis is caused by an underlying infection.[2] Explanations for why patients with sepsis remain culture negative can be early administration of broad-spectrum antibiotics before obtaining cultures, misdiagnosis, and lack of specific testing for the infecting bacteria.[35] Many retrospective studies about culture-negative sepsis include nonseptic patients,[35] and this is in part due to false-positive SIRS or qSOFA criteria, which further complicates the results and confounds the ability to draw meaningful conclusions. Because recommendations for the treatment of suspected sepsis is broad-spectrum antibiotics,[36] many nonseptic patients receive unnecessary antibiotic treatment. There is a desire to provide more targeted initial therapy because of growing concern of increasing resistance in bacteria.[35] It is hard to

quantify the likelihood that bacteremia develops into sepsis because bacteremia is a routine occurrence from gum insult from normal dental hygiene or even simple scrapes or cuts.

Blood cultures in the setting of PJI are at times collected but are not used in the PJI diagnostic criteria (Table 5). Studies have found that the presence of positive blood culture at the time of PJI diagnosis resulted in decreased rates of successfully treating the infected joint.[37] The development of PJI from bacteremia heavily depends on the pathogen[38] with *S aureus*, beta-hemolytic streptococci, and *Streptococcus viridians* associated with higher risks of infection, whereas *E coli* and coagulase-negative staphylococci bacteremia rarely leads to PJI.[38] A study by Honkanen and colleagues[38] showed that 7% of bacteremia episodes resulted in PJI. Patients with PJI who also have positive blood cultures are found to have lower success rates when treated with debridement, antibiotics, and implant retention (DAIR),[39] and it is recommended that these patients undergo a 2-stage approach for treatment.

Sepsis may occur in patients who have undergone TJA under many different circumstances. A patient with a TJA in place may develop sepsis from a completely separate cause, such as ruptured diverticulitis or appendix or a diabetic foot infection. Treatment of infectious conditions in the patient who has undergone TJA should involve quick delivery of IV antibiotics to prevent seeding of the joint. The length of time in which these patients should be treated with IV antibiotics is unknown, but studies have found that shorter and longer periods of treatment resulted in no significant difference in treatment outcomes.[40]

Patients whi have undergone TJA may also develop sepsis during or after surgery to remove the infected joint. If a tourniquet is used during removal of an infected TKA, the tourniquet release may initiate sepsis as the bacteria confined to the occluded vasculature of the limb are released into the systemic circulation. Blood loss is particularly high when infected THA is removed, and this may make a patient more susceptible to the sequalae of infection.[41] The surgeon and anesthesiologist must be aware of the risk for acute sepsis after removal of the infected joint; this should be treated with continued antibiotics, fluid resuscitation, blood product resuscitation, coagulopathy monitoring, and ICU admission when required. Risk of mortality in these patients is high, particularly when they are older than 80 years.[42] Patients with multiple infected joints, termed

Table 5
Major and Minor periprosthetic joint infection criteria

Major Criteria[a] (at least 1 of the following)				
Two positive cultures of the same organism				
A sinus tract or hollow cavity communicating with the arthroplasty				
Minor Criteria				Score
Preoperative diagnosis[b]	Serum		Elevated CRP or D-dimer	2
			Elevated ESR	1
	Synovial		Elevated synovial WBC or positive leukocyte	3
			Esterase test	
			Positive alpha-defensin	3
			Elevated synovial PMN (%)	2
			Elevated synovial CRP	1
Intraoperative diagnosis[c]				Score
	Preoperative Score (from above)			-
	Positive histology			3
	Positive purulence			3
	Single positive culture			2

Abbreviations: CRP, C-reactive protein; ESR, erythrocyte sedimentation rate; PMN, polymorponuclear cells; WBC, white blood cell.
  [a] PJI is diagnosed if at least 1 major criterion is met.
  [b] Preoperative minor criteria score ≥ 6 is an infection, 2 to 5 is a potential infection, 0 to 1 is no infection.
  [c] If there is a dry tap or inconclusive preoperative score, then use intraoperative diagnosis. Score greater than 6, infection; 4 to 5, inconclusive; ≤3, no infection.
  Data from BMC Musculoskeletal Disorders.

asynchronous infections, are also at high risk for sepsis and mortality.[43] These patients should be treated with great care by the surgeon, and discussion with the ICU should be made before surgery in case transfer is necessary.

Case reports
There are little data available on the diagnosis of sepsis in the patients who has undergone TJA, but several case reports have been published on the topic. Roth and colleagues[44] followed a 71-year-old insulin-dependent diabetic woman who received a left TKA for osteoarthritis. Before hospital admission, the patient developed a UTI that was being treated with ciprofloxacin. The postoperative course was initially unremarkable, but by postoperative day 9 necrotic tissue developed around the surgical site. The diseased tissue led to an early revision with complete removal of the prosthesis and insertion of a gentamycin-containing antibiotic spacer. Swabs taken intraoperatively found *S aureus* (resistant to only vancomycin) to be the cause of the infection within the knee, which then eventually spread to both shoulders. Despite adequate treatment with IV vancomycin, the patient

developed septic shock leading to an arthroscopic debridement of the knee and both shoulders with local lavage and instillation of vancomycin. The patient initially responded to treatment at secondary sites, but then her condition worsened to the point where above knee amputation was required as a lifesaving measure.

Krijnen and Wuisman[45] described 2 patients who became septic from an infection related to a previously placed THA. The first case describes a 63-year-old woman who had both left and right THAs 4.5 and 8 years prior, respectively. The patient described the pain starting in the right groin and radiating to the knee 18 months before admittance. The second case describes a 77-year-old woman who underwent a left THA 12 years prior. She had previously undergone revision 10 years after the THA due to implant loosening. One year after this, her right hip underwent THA leading to a deep wound infection. Surgical debridement and removal of the implant were performed but did not eradicate the infection. Both patients developed sepsis after multiple failed surgical attempts to control infection, necessitating hemipelvectomy for source control. Both patients were infection free after the hemipelvectomy but required a wheelchair (case 1) or maximal assistance (case 2) for long-term mobility.

Sepsis prophylaxis and treatment during and after surgery

Sepsis is a rare but deadly complication in patients who have undergone TJA with a 32-fold increase in mortality rates.[33] It is difficult to diagnose sepsis in the postoperative period because there are many normal findings in the postoperative patient, such as increased inflammatory markers and hypotension, which overlap with the diagnosis of early sepsis. Early stages of sepsis are likely to develop into severe sepsis or septic shock if not rapidly treated, making perioperative evaluation of organ function and an accurate determination of the present history of illness crucial.

Perioperative infection rates can be decreased in patients undergoing TJA by following well-established guidelines. The administration of prophylactic antibiotics before the surgical incision is a well-established practice shown to decrease the risk of surgical site infection.[20] Other common operating room practices such as proper skin preparation, limiting operating room traffic, and the use of aseptic wound closure techniques can decrease the risk of infection.[20] Proper wound care plays an important role in preventing postoperative infections. There are multiple options available for postoperative wound management to include the placement of a silver-impregnated occlusive dressing or the use of an incisional negative pressure dressing in patients who are at high risk for the development of a surgical site infection.[46] The potential for acute sepsis in the perioperative period of the surgical arthroplasty patient is quite low. There is a trend in the United States for TJA to be performed in the outpatient setting with many procedures now being performed in ambulatory surgery centers.[47] These centers are focused on providing surgical procedures where the patient can return home the same day and dose not have many of the services offered by a full-service hospital to include ICU beds. This is not an issue for most patients who have a joint replacement, but the surgeon may consider performing TJA in patients who are at high risk for sepsis in a facility that offers critical care services.

SUMMARY

Sepsis is a potentially fatal condition with an increasing incidence over the past several decades. There is limited literature available to guide the clinician in regard to sepsis in the patient who has undergone TJA. The few case reports reviewed in this article reveal the life-altering consequences that sepsis can have on patients who have undergone TJA. The development of infection, and subsequent sepsis, is best to be avoided by numerous perioperative practices, including appropriate patient selection and surgical optimization, patient education on proper wound care technique, detecting early signs of UTI or lung infections, and following proper sterile operating room protocols. Some patients may not be appropriate candidates to undergo arthroplasty if they have multiple predisposing factors for PJI. These common risk factors include obesity, diabetes mellitus, tobacco usage, and a weakened immune system. If a patient becomes septic in the setting of TJA, treatment with broad-spectrum antibiotics within 1 hour of diagnoses is crucial and IV fluids should be administered within 30 minutes. The lack of current literature on sepsis among the TJA population makes exact recommendations for treatment difficult, but the broader literature on sepsis can provide guidance for the physician tasked with treating the patient with this difficult problem.

CLINICS CARE POINTS

- Orthopedic surgeons should be aware of the potential for sepsis in patients with PJI.
- The definition of sepsis has changed over the years, but the most used designation is defined by SIRS criteria.
- Patients with positive SIRS criteria should be carefully and comprehensively evaluated for sepsis.
- Sepsis on presentation to the emergency room in a patient with PJI should be treated with aggressive antibiotics and IV fluids. Intensive care monitoring may be required.
- If necessary, joint aspiration to diagnose PJI may need to be performed after antibiotics are started to treat sepsis.
- Surgeons and anesthesiologists should carefully monitor patients for signs of sepsis during admission and treatment of PJI.
- Patients may require hemodynamic support and ICU treatment if sepsis occurs during PJI treatment.

DISCLOSURE

Please see the AAOS Web site for relevant disclosures.

REFERENCES

1. Ulrich SD, Seyler TM, Bennett D, et al. Total hip arthroplasties: What are the reasons for revision? Int Orthopaedics 2008;32(5). https://doi.org/10.1007/s00264-007-0364-3.
2. Mingle D. The Evolving Definition of Sepsis. Int Clin Pathol J 2016;2(6). https://doi.org/10.15406/icpjl.2016.02.00063.
3. Singh JA, Yu S, Chen L, et al. Rates of Total Joint Replacement in the United States: Future Projections to 2020–2040 Using the National Inpatient Sample. J Rheumatol 2019;46(9). https://doi.org/10.3899/jrheum.170990.
4. Kurtz S, Ong K, Lau E, et al. Projections of Primary and Revision Hip and Knee Arthroplasty in the United States from 2005 to 2030. J Bone Joint Surg 2007;89(4). https://doi.org/10.2106/JBJS.F.00222.
5. Tande AJ, Patel R. Prosthetic Joint Infection. Clin Microbiol Rev 2014;27(2). https://doi.org/10.1128/CMR.00111-13.
6. Hernández-Vaquero D, Fernández-Fairen M, Torres A, et al. Treatment of Periprosthetic Infections: An Economic Analysis. Scientific World J 2013;2013. https://doi.org/10.1155/2013/821650.
7. Guan H, Xu C, Fu J, et al. Diagnostic criteria of periprosthetic joint infection: a prospective study protocol to validate the feasibility of the 2018 new definition for Chinese patients. BMC Musculoskelet Disord 2019;20(1). https://doi.org/10.1186/s12891-019-2941-1.
8. Parvizi J, Aggarwal V, Rasouli M. Periprosthetic joint infection: Current concept. Indian J Orthopaedics 2013;47(1). https://doi.org/10.4103/0019-5413.106884.
9. Hofmann AA, Goldberg T, Tanner AM, et al. Treatment of Infected Total Knee Arthroplasty Using an Articulating Spacer. Clin Orthopaedics Relat Res 2005;430. https://doi.org/10.1097/01.blo.0000149241.77924.01.
10. Frank JM, Kayupov E, Moric M, et al. The Mark Coventry, MD, Award: Oral Antibiotics Reduce Reinfection After Two-Stage Exchange: A Multicenter, Randomized Controlled Trial. Clin Orthopaedics Relat Res 2017;475(1). https://doi.org/10.1007/s11999-016-4890-4.
11. Jacobi J. Pathophysiology of sepsis. Am J Health-System Pharm 2002;59(suppl_1). https://doi.org/10.1093/ajhp/59.suppl_1.S3.
12. Torio CM, Andrews RM.National Inpatient Hospital Costs: The Most Expensive Conditions by Payer. 2013. Available at: https://www.ncbi.nlm.nih.gov/books/NBK368492/.
13. Martin GS, Mannino DM, Eaton S, et al. The Epidemiology of Sepsis in the United States from 1979 through 2000. New Engl J Med 2003;348(16). https://doi.org/10.1056/NEJMoa022139.
14. Wang T, Derhovanessian A, de Cruz S, et al. Subsequent Infections in Survivors of Sepsis. J Intensive Care Med 2014;29(2). https://doi.org/10.1177/0885066612467162.
15. Polat G, Ugan RA, Cadirci E, et al. Sepsis and Septic Shock: Current Treatment Strategies and New Approaches. The Eurasian J Med 2017;49(1). https://doi.org/10.5152/eurasianjmed.2017.17062.
16. Balk RA. Systemic inflammatory response syndrome (SIRS). Virulence 2014;5(1). https://doi.org/10.4161/viru.27135.
17. Jones GR, Lowes JA. The systemic inflammatory response syndrome as a predictor of bacteraemia and outcome from sepsis. QJM 1996;89(7). https://doi.org/10.1093/qjmed/89.7.515.
18. Gul F, Arslantas MK, Cinel I, et al. Changing Definitions of Sepsis. Turk J Anesth Reanimation 2017;45(3). https://doi.org/10.5152/TJAR.2017.93753.
19. Dykes LA, Heintz SJ, Heintz BH, et al. Contrasting qSOFA and SIRS Criteria for Early Sepsis Identification in a Veteran Population. Fed Pract 2019;36(Suppl 2):S21–4.
20. Daines BK, Dennis DA, Amann S. Infection Prevention in Total Knee Arthroplasty. J Am Acad Orthopaedic Surgeons 2015;23(6). https://doi.org/10.5435/JAAOS-D-12-00170.
21. Zitek T, Bourne M, Raber J, et al. Blood Culture Results and Overtreatment Associated With the Use of a 1-Hour Sepsis Bundle. J Emerg Med 2020;59(5). https://doi.org/10.1016/j.jemermed.2020.06.055.
22. Fitzpatrick F, Tarrant C, Hamilton V, et al. Sepsis and antimicrobial stewardship: two sides of the same coin. BMJ Qual Saf 2019;28(9). https://doi.org/10.1136/bmjqs-2019-009445.
23. Minderhoud TC, Spruyt C, Huisman S, Oskam E, Schuit S, Levin MD. Microbiological outcomes and antibiotic overuse in Emergency Department patients with suspected sepsis. Neth J Med 2017;75(5):196–203.
24. Worapratya P, Wuthisuthimethawee P. Septic shock in the ER: diagnostic and management challenges. Open Access Emerg Med 2019;11. https://doi.org/10.2147/OAEM.S166086.
25. Almutary A, Althunayyan S, Alenazi K, et al. National Early Warning Score (NEWS) as Prognostic Triage Tool for Septic Patients. Infect Drug Resist 2020;13. https://doi.org/10.2147/IDR.S275390.
26. Morley PT. Early Fluid Management in Sepsis. Crit Care Med 2018;46(2). https://doi.org/10.1097/CCM.0000000000002880.
27. Chang R, Holcomb JB. Choice of Fluid Therapy in the Initial Management of Sepsis, Severe Sepsis, and Septic Shock. Shock 2016;46(1). https://doi.org/10.1097/SHK.0000000000000577.
28. Bennett SR. Sepsis in the intensive care unit. Surgery (Oxford) 2015;33(11). https://doi.org/10.1016/j.mpsur.2015.08.002.

29. Martínez ML, Plata-Menchaca EP, Ruiz-Rodríguez JC, et al. An approach to antibiotic treatment in patients with sepsis. J Thorac Dis 2020;12(3). https://doi.org/10.21037/jtd.2020.01.47.

30. Goh GS, Parvizi J. Think Twice before Prescribing Antibiotics for That Swollen Knee: The Influence of Antibiotics on the Diagnosis of Periprosthetic Joint Infection. Antibiotics 2021;10(2). https://doi.org/10.3390/antibiotics10020114.

31. Lockhart GC, Hanin J, Micek ST, et al. Pathogen-Negative Sepsis—An Opportunity for Antimicrobial Stewardship. Open Forum Infect Dis 2019;6(10). https://doi.org/10.1093/ofid/ofz397.

32. Nasser S. The incidence of sepsis after total hip replacement arthroplasty. Semin Arthroplasty 1994;5(4):153–9.

33. Bohl DD, Sershon RA, Fillingham YA, et al. Incidence, Risk Factors, and Sources of Sepsis Following Total Joint Arthroplasty. J Arthroplasty 2016;31(12). https://doi.org/10.1016/j.arth.2016.05.031.

34. Nannan Panday RS, Lammers EMJ, Alam N, et al. An overview of positive cultures and clinical outcomes in septic patients: a sub-analysis of the Prehospital Antibiotics Against Sepsis (PHANTASi) trial. Crit Care 2019;23(1). https://doi.org/10.1186/s13054-019-2431-8.

35. Thorndike J, Kollef MH. Culture-negative sepsis. Curr Opin Crit Care 2020;26(5). https://doi.org/10.1097/MCC.0000000000000751.

36. Rhodes A, Evans LE, Alhazzani W, et al. Surviving Sepsis Campaign: International Guidelines for Management of Sepsis and Septic Shock: 2016. Intensive Care Med 2017;43(3). https://doi.org/10.1007/s00134-017-4683-6.

37. Klement MR, Siddiqi A, Rock JM, et al. Positive Blood Cultures in Periprosthetic Joint Infection Decrease Rate of Treatment Success. The J Arthroplasty 2018;33(1). https://doi.org/10.1016/j.arth.2017.08.034.

38. Honkanen M, Jämsen E, Karppelin M, et al. Periprosthetic Joint Infections as a Consequence of Bacteremia. Open Forum Infect Dis 2019;6(6). https://doi.org/10.1093/ofid/ofz218.

39. Kuo F-C, Goswami K, Klement MR, et al. Positive Blood Cultures Decrease the Treatment Success in Acute Hematogenous Periprosthetic Joint Infection Treated With Debridement, Antibiotics, and Implant Retention. The J Arthroplasty 2019;34(12). https://doi.org/10.1016/j.arth.2019.06.053.

40. Havey TC, Fowler RA, Daneman N. Duration of antibiotic therapy for bacteremia: a systematic review and meta-analysis. Crit Care 2011;15(6). https://doi.org/10.1186/cc10545.

41. Lenguerrand E, Whitehouse MR, Beswick AD, et al. Risk factors associated with revision for prosthetic joint infection following knee replacement: an observational cohort study from England and Wales. Lancet Infect Dis 2019;19(6). https://doi.org/10.1016/S1473-3099(18)30755-2.

42. Yilmaz E, Poell A, Baecker H, et al. Poor outcome of octogenarians admitted to ICU due to periprosthetic joint infections: a retrospective cohort study. BMC Musculoskelet Disord 2020;21(1). https://doi.org/10.1186/s12891-020-03331-0.

43. Gausden EB, Pagnano MW, Perry KI, et al. Synchronous Periprosthetic Joint Infections: High Mortality, Reinfection, and Reoperation. J Arthroplasty 2021. https://doi.org/10.1016/j.arth.2021.05.010.

44. Venbrocks R, Lange M, Roth A, et al. Overwhelming septic infection with a multi-resistant Staphylococcus aureus (MRSA) after total knee replacement. Arch Orthopaedic Trauma Surg 2003;123(8). https://doi.org/10.1007/s00402-003-0535-7.

45. Krijnen MR, Wuisman PIJM. Emergency hemipelvectomy as a result of uncontrolled infection after total hip arthroplasty. The J Arthroplasty 2004;19(6). https://doi.org/10.1016/j.arth.2004.01.008.

46. Doman DM, Young AM, Buller LT, et al. Comparison of Surgical Site Complications With Negative Pressure Wound Therapy vs Silver Impregnated Dressing in High-Risk Total Knee Arthroplasty Patients: A Matched Cohort Study. J Arthroplasty 2021. https://doi.org/10.1016/j.arth.2021.05.030.

47. Bert JM, Hooper J, Moen S. Outpatient Total Joint Arthroplasty. Curr Rev Musculoskelet Med 2017;10(4). https://doi.org/10.1007/s12178-017-9451-2.

Compartment Syndrome After Hip and Knee Arthroplasty

Aresh Sepehri, MD, MSc,
Lisa C. Howard, MD, MHSc, FRCSC,
Michael E. Neufeld, MD, MSc, FRCSC,
Bassam A. Masri, MD, FRCSC*

KEYWORDS

- Acute compartment syndrome • Total joint arthroplasty • Fasciotomy

---

KEY POINTS

- Acute compartment syndrome is a rare postoperative complication of hip and knee arthroplasties, which can be difficult to diagnose, given the natural postoperative course with regards to pain and multimodal pain management techniques
- Acute compartment syndrome is a surgical emergency with fasciotomy of the involved compartments being the mainstay of treatment
- Meticulous hemostasis during the procedure, careful patient positioning particularly in the lateral position, and limiting prolonged postoperative epidural infusions should be practiced to limit ACS risk

---

INTRODUCTION

Acute compartment syndrome (ACS) of the lower extremity is an orthopedic emergency, which occurs when elevated pressures within a myofascial compartment lead to reduced blood flow and subsequently inadequate tissue perfusion.[1,2] Prolonged intracompartmental pressure elevation can lead to necrosis of the soft tissues within a compartment, including muscle and neurovascular structures. ACS is associated with significant patient morbidity and a delayed diagnosis can result in permanent disability. Early recognition is paramount in the management of ACS, as timely diagnosis and fasciotomy are imperative in preventing the sequelae of compartment syndrome.[3]

ACS has been well documented after the traumatic orthopedic injuries such as crush injuries or long bone fractures.[4] Fasciotomies are frequently performed prophylactically in the setting of vascular injury as reperfusion syndrome after repair is a known risk factor for compartment syndrome.[5] In contrast, ACS after total hip or knee arthroplasty is encountered very infrequently with literature on the topic limited to case reports and case series. As a result, there is often a delay in diagnosis and management, which can have dramatic impacts on patient functional outcomes. This article reviews the literature on the etiology, diagnosis, and management of compartment syndrome after hip and knee arthroplasties.

COMMON ETIOLOGIES OF ACUTE COMPARTMENT SYNDROME IN HIP AND KNEE ARTHROPLASTIES

Anticoagulation

Postoperative anticoagulation has been reported as a risk factor for postoperative

---

Department of Orthopaedics, University of British Columbia, 3rd Floor, 2775 Laurel Street, Vancouver, British Columbia V5Z 1M9, Canada
* Corresponding author. Department of Orthopaedics, University of British Columbia, Complex Joint Reconstruction Clinic, Gordon & Leslie Diamond Health Care Centre, 3rd Floor, 2775 Laurel Street, Vancouver, British Columbia V5Z 1M9, Canada.
E-mail address: bas.masri@ubc.ca

hematoma leading to ACS.[6] Nadeem and colleagues[7] in their retrospective case series of 2 total hip and 1 total knee arthroplasties describe 3 instances of ACS due to a thigh hematoma. All patients were on preoperative or postoperative anticoagulation: one was receiving prophylactic anticoagulation with heparin, one was on preoperative anticoagulation due to stroke and underwent bridging therapy before surgery, and one was recently transitioned from heparin to therapeutic warfarin postoperatively for a diagnosed deep vein thrombosis (DVT). The development of ACS occurred in the late postoperative period with the diagnosis made between postoperative days 3 and 6 in all patients. In the setting of anticoagulation, large hematoma formation can occur without specific vessel injury.[8,9] All patients underwent a fasciotomy and hematoma evacuation. Only 1 patient was found to have an identifiable vascular injury. If concerns for vascular injury are present, a computed tomography angiography (CTA) can be performed preoperatively for surgical planning purposes.

Vascular Injury

Injury to the arterial or venous vessels can lead to compartment syndrome through a variety of mechanisms. Venous insufficiency, either due to thrombus formation[10] or direct injury with occlusion, has been reported as a cause of compartment syndrome after total knee arthroplasty.[11,12] Although venous hemorrhage will often tamponade before significant increases in compartment pressures, bleeding from an arterial injury can result in large hematoma formation and subsequent ACS. Prolonged ischemia from a popliteal, femoral, or external iliac artery injury and the associated reperfusion syndrome after repair or reconstruction can be associated with ACS.[5,13] Although anticoagulation may increase the risk of hematoma formation, particularly in the late postoperative period as outlined earlier, in the case series of 7 total knee arthroplasty patients with postoperative ACS by Haggis and colleagues,[11] only 1 of 4 cases associated with an identified vascular injury were receiving anticoagulation at the time of diagnosis.

Multiple case reports[8,14,15] have discussed the increased risk of hematoma formation with the anterior approach to total hip replacement, which resulted in ACS requiring fasciotomies. Ligation of branches of the lateral circumflex femoral artery is required to successfully access the hip joint. Incomplete ligation or unrecognized injury can result in hematoma formation of the anterior thigh compartment leading to ACS. However, acute postoperative bleeding and hematoma formation resulting in ACS are published using the lateral and posterior approaches to the hip as well, and are not specific to the anterior approach.[16]

Intraoperative Positioning

Well limb compartment syndrome has been documented in prolonged procedures where the patient is placed lateral decubitus.[17] In a cohort of healthy volunteers, it has been demonstrated that the dependent limb in the lateral decubitus position can have elevated compartment pressures up to 240 mm Hg in the anterior tibial compartment.[18] Prolonged increased compartment pressures, even in the absence of trauma, can mimic crush injuries, resulting in intracompartmental edema and subsequent ACS. Kumar and colleagues[19] described 4 cases of gluteal compartment syndrome following arthroplasty, of which 2 cases occurred in the well limb following lateral decubitus positioning for total hip arthroplasty. Both cases had prolonged procedure times of 2 hours and 20 minutes and 3 hours and prolonged patient positioning in the lateral position was attributed as the cause of ACS. In a literature review by Lasanianos and colleagues,[16] of 22 ACS cases following total hip arthroplasty, 16 occurred in the contralateral gluteal compartment. Although the operating table and positioning protocol were not specifically reported, this emphasizes the need for careful patient positioning with adequate padding under the gluteal region, in addition to the padding routinely placed under bony prominences.

DIAGNOSIS

The diagnosis of ACS should be based on clinical assessment when able (Table 1).[2,20] Inspection of the limb may find a swollen compartment that is firm to palpation. Patients often complain of pain that is out of proportion to the postoperative course or pain unrelieved by increasing amounts of analgesia, particularly opioid medications. Palpation of the compartments and passive stretch of the muscles and tendons within the compartment increase intracompartment pressures, causing increased pain during assessment. The earliest signs of increased compartment pressures are sensory deficits and paresthesia. The sensory axons are more vulnerable to ischemia than motor axons, with motor deficits, or paralysis, being a later finding of ACS.[21]

In the later stages of ACS, pain can be absent as prolonged ischemia can lead to nerve

Table 1
Diagnosis of compartment syndrome

Acute Compartment Syndrome Diagnosis	
Clinical Examination	• Pain out proportion, paresthesia, paralysis, firm compartments on palpation, pain with passive stretch
Compartment Pressure Measurements	• Absolute pressure >30 mm Hg • ΔP <30 mm Hg (diastolic blood pressure – compartment pressure)
Serum and Urine Biomarkers	• Elevated creatine kinase, myoglobinuria

necrosis and hypoesthesia. Systemic markers of muscle necrosis can be measured including myoglobinuria and creatine kinase. Compartment pressures that are elevated above the systolic blood pressure can result in pulselessness, although this is a rare finding and not a requirement for ACS diagnosis. This can lead to pallor of the skin and a cool limb compared to the contralateral side. Conversely, pulselessness should be considered a sign of a primary vascular injury and prompt emergent investigation and management.

In the vast majority of elective arthroplasty patients, the patients are alert and competent to perform a clinical assessment. However, prolonged postoperative regional anesthesia can make sensory and motor examinations unreliable.[16,22,23] Kumar and colleagues[19] reported 4 cases of compartment syndrome with delayed diagnosis attributed to postoperative epidural infusions. Kumar and colleagues suggested that epidural infusions should be titrated to allow motor function, decreasing postoperative immobilization and allowing partial sensory function and examination. Similarly, Haggis and colleagues[11] found that in 5 patients who were diagnosed with ACS and received an epidural infusion after total knee arthroplasty, 3 patients were only diagnosed after the epidural infusion was discontinued.

In cases where ACS is suspected but a clinical diagnosis cannot be made reliably, compartment pressure monitoring should be performed. Needle manometers can be inserted into the compartment and measured in mm Hg.[24] Normal compartment pressures range from 0 to 8 mm Hg, although no studies have evaluated "normal" compartment pressure after hip or knee replacement in patients with no signs or symptoms of compartment syndrome. A threshold value of 30 mm Hg has been used for fasciotomy indication, as prior studies have shown that pressures under this value can be treated without fasciotomy with no sequelae.[24] Of note, in a case series of tibial shaft fractures,

elevated compartment pressures, even above 40 mm Hg, in the absence of symptoms were not associated with the long-term functional sequelae seen in diagnosed ACS.[25] Rather than an absolute threshold value, some have advocated calculating the difference between diastolic blood pressure and compartment pressures, where ACS is diagnosed when compartment pressures are within 30 mm Hg.[26,27]

There is significant variability in the technique for compartment pressure measurements that results in low interobserver reliability.[28] Pressures within a compartment vary based on location.[29] Although pressure measurement sites are well defined in fracture care, this is not the case in joint arthroplasty. Ultimately routine pressure measurements are not recommended and should be reserved for cases where clinical suspicion is high and ACS cannot be ruled out by clinical examination. Furthermore, although noninvasive methods for determining compartment pressures have been proposed, such as near-infrared spectroscopy and laser Doppler flowmetry, there are limited literature and guidelines for diagnosis and indications for these techniques.[30]

MANAGEMENT

When compartment syndrome is suspected, the initial management should involve removing all circumferential dressings, such as a tensor bandage dressing. Removal of circumferential soft dressings has been found to decrease compartment pressures by 10% to 20%.[31] The limb should be elevated to heart level to maintain perfusion pressure within vessels but minimize gravity-dependent swelling and edema.

However, if the clinical examination does not improve expeditiously with the aforementioned conservative management, the definitive treatment involves fasciotomy of the involved limb. The time to fasciotomy is a significant predictor in patient outcomes and fasciotomy should not be significantly delayed with the aforementioned nonoperative management.[32] Although the threshold for permanent muscle damage was reported after 8 hours,[33] muscle necrosis has been observed in animal models after as little as 4 hours of ischemia.[34] If fasciotomy was performed within 12 hours, 68% of patients made a full functional recovery, compared to 8% if performed after 12 hours.[3]

There is controversy in the optimal management of patients with a delayed diagnosis of compartment syndrome. Once myonecrosis and nerve cell death occur, fasciotomy will provide little benefit in terms of functional recovery. Late fasciotomy was associated with increased infection complications and had worse outcomes than those treated nonoperatively, which were associated with muscle contractures.[35–37] However, these studies were in trauma and crush injury patients rather than an arthroplasty population. Significant rhabdomyolysis with systemic symptoms, in particular severe acute kidney injury, is a consideration in treatment decision-making for delayed fasciotomy. Even though there may be no musculoskeletal functional benefit to late fasciotomy, removal of necrotic muscle will decrease the serum electrolyte imbalances and muscle enzyme levels, such as creatine kinase, and can help prevent further kidney injury. These decisions need to be made on a case-by-case basis based on collaboration with medical colleagues.

ACS following a total joint replacement can be a result of tissue trauma and edema associated with the operation. **Fig. 1** demonstrates a 59-year-old male who underwent a total knee replacement. No intraoperative concerns were noted. Overnight following the procedure, the patient developed increasing pain and swelling in the anterior thigh compartment. The compartment was firm to palpation. Owing to concerns for an expanding hematoma or vascular injury, a CTA was performed. No vascular injury was identified but pronounced swelling and increased size of the anterior compartment compared to the contralateral limb were noted (see **Fig. 1C**). The patient was taken emergently to the operating room for fasciotomy, where it was noted there was significant generalized swelling and edema in the quadriceps muscle.

Notably, ACS after arthroplasty can frequently have a specific pathology resulting in increased compartment pressures. Fasciotomy remains the mainstay of management for ACS. However, surgeons should be vigilant in addressing the underlying pathology simultaneously. Frequently, ACS can be caused by an expanding hematoma because of nonspecific bleeding or identifiable vessel injury. In the setting of hematoma formation without specific vessel injury, Hogerzeil and colleagues[8] reported using topical tranexamic acid as an adjunct, in addition to fasciotomy and hematoma evacuation, to decrease hematoma recurrence. Although major arterial injury is rare in total joint arthroplasty, cited around 0.13%,[38] if identified, prompt vascular surgery consultation is required. In the setting of a dysvascular limb, open surgical revascularization is required. In the setting of ACS with arterial injury and a well-perfused limb, open ligation of vessels can frequently be performed during the fasciotomy. Nadeem and colleagues[7] described a total hip replacement case performed with a posterior approach, with postoperative thigh ACS. A fasciotomy of the thigh was performed in conjunction with hematoma evacuation of the posterior thigh compartment. Ongoing hemorrhage was identified intraoperatively, and a vascular surgeon

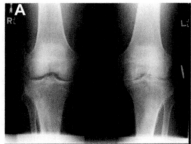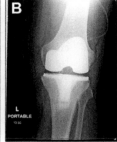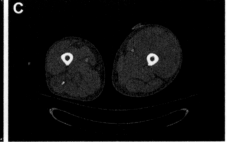

Fig. 1. A 59-year-old male with tricompartmental osteoarthritis of the left knee (A) who undergoes an uncomplicated total knee arthroplasty (B). Overnight, the patient developed significant pain and swelling in the anterior thigh compartment. A CTA scan was performed to rule out a vascular injury or expanding hematoma. No vascular injury was found, but there was pronounced swelling and increased size of the anterior compartment compared to the contralateral limb (C). The patient underwent thigh fasciotomy. Intraoperatively, it was noted there was significant generalized swelling and edema in the quadriceps muscle with no other underlying pathology.

was consulted. Ultimately, the profunda femoris artery was ligated through an anterior approach by the vascular team. Intraoperative angiography with endovascular procedures for hemorrhage control is also described.[38,39]

Management of ACS of the gluteal compartment due to prolonged compression is currently under debate. Lachiewicz and colleagues[40] reported 6 cases of contralateral gluteal ACS in patients undergoing total hip arthroplasty in the lateral position. The ACS was attributed to patient positioning. Although all patients were diagnosed with compartment syndrome and rhabdomyolysis, only the first patient underwent fasciotomy following compartment pressure assessment with a needle manometer, measuring 50 mm Hg. The remaining 5 patients were treated nonoperatively with medical management for rhabdomyolysis. Myoglobinuria resolved in all patients. No motor deficits were present at 2 weeks, although 2 patients had ongoing paresthesia in the sciatic nerve distribution 2 years postoperatively.

FASCIOTOMY TECHNIQUE OF THE LOWER EXTREMITY

Gluteal compartment syndrome is a relatively rare site for ACS in the trauma population, but has been reported after prolonged compression of the compartment due to immobilization, as is seen in arthroplasty patients placed in the lateral position for prolonged periods.[41,42] Clinical examination often elicits sciatic nerve palsy symptoms, as the nerve is located underneath the gluteal muscles and is fixed between the piriformis and obturator tendons. Significant gluteal swelling can result in nerve compression. It should be noted that an expanding hematoma can cause sciatic nerve compression and injury in the absence of ACS. A progressive acute postoperative sciatic nerve palsy with concern for a hematoma is a surgical emergency in itself even without ACS. The gluteal region involves 3 compartments: tensor fascia latae, gluteus maximus, and gluteus medius/minimus. Fasciotomy release should include all 3 compartments. This is often accomplished through a Kocher-Langenbeck, particularly if a posterior approach to the hip was performed, or a modified Gibson approach. A Kocher-Langenbeck approach is performed through a curvilinear skin incision starting lateral to the posterior superior iliac spine extending anteriorly and distally to the greater trochanter, and distally along the lateral femur to the insertion of the gluteus maximus muscle. A sciatic nerve neurolysis is frequently performed simultaneously.

The thigh is divided into the following 3 compartments: (1) the anterior compartment includes the quadriceps and sartorius muscles and femoral nerve; (2) the posterior compartment includes the hamstring muscles and sciatic nerve; and (3) the adductor compartment includes the adductor muscles and obturator nerve. Fasciotomy is performed with a lateral approach to the femur to access the anterior and posterior compartments.[43,44] Dissection through fascia latae provides access to the anterior compartment. The vastus lateralis is elevated off the lateral intermuscular septum, which can be incised releasing the posterior compartment. It is hypothesized that the adductor compartment is not frequently involved in ACS of the thigh and it is debated whether a formal release of the medial compartment is required in all cases. Intraoperative compartment pressure measurement can be performed after release of the anterior and posterior thigh compartments to aid in decision making. The adductor compartment is released through a separate medial incision directly overlaying the adductor muscles.

There are 4 compartments in the lower leg: the anterior, lateral, deep posterior, and superficial posterior compartments. The more common fasciotomy technique of the lower leg is the 2-incision approach.[45,46] An anterolateral incision is performed anterior to the fibula, approximately over the intermuscular septum. Once this septum is identified, the anterior and lateral compartments can be released, taking care to preserve the superficial peroneal nerve distally which exists the fascia in the distal third of the leg coursing anteriorly. A second posteromedial incision is performed posterior to the palpable edge of the tibia. This provides access to the superficial posterior compartment which can be released. To gain access to the deep posterior compartment, the soleus must be elevated off the posteromedial edge of the tibia. The deep posterior fascia can then be released. The posterior tibial neurovascular bundle runs between the deep and superficial compartments and should be preserved.

OUTCOMES OF ACUTE COMPARTMENT SYNDROME IN TOTAL JOINT ARTHROPLASTY

Outcomes of ACS after total joint arthroplasty are often poor. This can be attributed to several factors including delayed diagnosis, advanced age and comorbidities in the patient population, and the etiology of ACS. The average time to diagnosis in the case series by Haggis and colleagues[11] was 58 hours postoperatively, with 5 of 7 eligible patients have permanent foot drop. Total knee arthroplasty can be quite painful in the early postoperative period, making the diagnosis of ACS challenging in this patient population and further delaying management. Prolonged epidural anesthetic has frequently been described as a contributing factor to delayed diagnosis. In complicated cases with prolonged operative time, such as revision cases, it has been suggested that epidural anesthetic be avoided completely.[47]

In addition, because of the advanced age of the arthroplasty patient population, there are frequently associated comorbidities including obesity and peripheral vascular disease, both of which were associated with ACS.[48] When ACS is a result of vascular injury, wound healing and tissue perfusion of both the arthroplasty surgical site and fasciotomy site are of significant concern. In a case series by Vegari and colleagues,[49] 5 cases were associated with vascular injury. Three of these cases sustained sequelae of infection and nonhealing surgical incision sites, one requiring an above knee amputation due to periprosthetic infection.

SUMMARY

Although a rare complication in the total joint replacement population, early diagnosis and prompt definitive management of ACS are paramount in preventing the significant morbidity associated with compartment syndrome. Given the painful postoperative period following joint replacement, the diagnosis of compartment syndrome can be difficult. Surgeons should maintain a high clinical suspicion of ACS in patients with risk factors, including obesity, receiving postoperative epidural infusion, and prolonged operative time. Furthermore, emphasis on limiting risk factors for ACS should be practiced, including meticulous hemostasis, careful patient positioning, and limiting prolonged postoperative regional anesthesia when not required.

CLINICS CARE POINTS

- The diagnosis of ACS is based on clinical examination, with compartment pressure measurements being limited to patients with an unreliable examination

- Expanding hematoma within a compartment can be due to anticoagulation or vascular injury, and should be addressed when undergoing fasciotomy

- In the setting of vascular injury, urgent vascular consultation should be obtained for concomitant open vascular repair or endovascular intervention

- Patient positioning during long operative cases, particularly in the lateral position for total hip arthroplasty, can result in compartment syndrome, particularly in the well leg or down leg.

- Management of gluteal compartment syndrome is controversial, with level 4 evidence demonstrating nonoperative management can lead to acceptable results.

DISCLOSURE

The authors have nothing to disclose.

REFERENCES

1. Guo J, Yin Y, Jin L, et al. Acute compartment syndrome: cause, diagnosis, and new viewpoint. Medicine (Baltimore) 2019;98(27):e16260.
2. Tiwari A, Haq AI, Myint F, et al. Acute compartment syndromes. Br J Surg 2002;89(4):397–412.
3. Sheridan GW, Matsen rFA. Fasciotomy in the treatment of the acute compartment syndrome. J Bone Joint Surg Am 1976;58(1):112.
4. McQueen MM, Gaston P, Court-Brown CM. Acute compartment syndrome. Who is at risk? J Bone Joint Surg Br 2000;82(2):200–3.
5. Lyden SP, Shortell CK, Illig KA. Reperfusion and compartment syndromes: strategies for prevention and treatment. Semin Vasc Surg 2001;14(2):107–13.
6. Hynson JM. Role of heparin in compartment syndrome. J Bone Joint Surg Am 2000;82(5):752–3.
7. Nadeem RD, Clift BA, Martindale JP, et al. Acute compartment syndrome of the thigh after joint replacement with anticoagulation. J Bone Joint Surg Br 1998;80(5):866–8.
8. Hogerzeil DP, Muradin I, Zwitser EW, et al. Acute compartment syndrome of the thigh following hip replacement by anterior approach in a patient using oral anticoagulants. World J Orthop 2017; 8(12):964–7.
9. Fleming RE Jr, Michelsen CB, Stinchfield FE. Sciatic paralysis. A complication of bleeding following hip surgery. J Bone Joint Surg Am 1979;61(1):37–9.
10. Rahm M, Probe R. Extensive deep venous thrombosis resulting in compartment syndrome of the thigh and leg. A case report. J Bone Joint Surg Am 1994;76(12):1854–7.

11. Haggis P, Yates P, Blakeway C, et al. Compartment syndrome following total knee arthroplasty. J Bone Joint Surg Br 2006;88-B(3):331–4.

12. Sánchez CA, Jara AB, Mariño J. Superficial femoral artery pseudoaneurysm, compartment syndrome, and deep vein thrombosis after total knee arthroplasty. Arthroplast Today 2020;6(2):227–30.

13. Pal A, Clarke JMF, Cameron AEP. Case series and literature review: popliteal artery injury following total knee replacement. Int J Surg 2010;8(6):430–5.

14. Elsorafy KR, Jm Stone A, Nicol SG. Acute compartment syndrome of the thigh 10 days following an elective primary total hip replacement. Ortop Traumatol Rehabil 2013;15(3):269–71.

15. Mai DD, MacDonald SJ, Bourne RB. Compartment syndrome of the right anterior thigh after primary total hip arthroplasty. Can J Surg 2000;43(3):226–7.

16. Lasanianos NG, Kanakaris NK, Roberts CS, et al. Compartment syndrome following lower limb arthroplasty: a review. Open Orthop J 2011;5:181–92.

17. Cascio BM, Buchowski JM, Frassica FJ. Well-limb compartment syndrome after prolonged lateral decubitus positioning. A report of two cases. J Bone Joint Surg Am 2004;86(9):2038–40.

18. Owen CA, Mubarak SJ, Hargens AR, et al. Intramuscular pressures with limb compression. N Engl J Med 1979;300(21):1169–72.

19. Kumar V, Saeed K, Panagopoulos A, et al. Gluteal compartment syndrome following joint arthroplasty under epidural anaesthesia: a report of 4 cases. J Orthop Surg (Hong Kong) 2007;15(1):113–7.

20. Via AG, Oliva F, Spoliti M, et al. Acute compartment syndrome. Muscles Ligaments Tendons J 2015;5(1):18–22.

21. Hofmeijer J, Franssen H, van Schelven LJ, et al. Why are sensory axons more vulnerable for ischemia than motor axons? PLoS One 2013;8(6):e67113.

22. Mar GJ, Barrington MJ, McGuirk BR. Acute compartment syndrome of the lower limb and the effect of postoperative analgesia on diagnosis. Br J Anaesth 2009;102(1):3–11.

23. Tang WM, Chiu KY. Silent compartment syndrome complicating total knee arthroplasty: continuous epidural anesthesia masked the pain. J Arthroplasty 2000;15(2):241–3.

24. Mubarak SJ, Owen CA, Hargens AR, et al. Acute compartment syndromes: diagnosis and treatment with the aid of the wick catheter. J Bone Joint Surg Am 1978;60(8):1091–5.

25. Triffitt PD, König D, Harper WM, et al. Compartment pressures after closed tibial shaft fracture. Their relation to functional outcome. J Bone Joint Surg Br 1992;74(2):195–8.

26. Whitesides TE, Haney TC, Morimoto K, et al. Tissue pressure measurements as a determinant for the need of fasciotomy. Clin Orthop Relat Res 1975;113:43–51.

27. McQueen MM, Court-Brown CM. Compartment monitoring in tibial fractures. The pressure threshold for decompression. J Bone Joint Surg Br 1996;78(1):99–104.

28. Nudel I, Dorfmann L, deBotton G. The compartment syndrome: is the intra-compartment pressure a reliable indicator for early diagnosis? Math Med Biol 2017;34(4):547–58.

29. Heckman MM, Whitesides TE Jr, Grewe SR, et al. Compartment pressure in association with closed tibial fractures. The relationship between tissue pressure, compartment, and the distance from the site of the fracture. J Bone Joint Surg Am 1994;76(9):1285–92.

30. Harvey EJ, Sanders DW, Shuler MS, et al. What's new in acute compartment syndrome? J Orthop Trauma 2012;26(12):699–702.

31. Garfin SR, Mubarak SJ, Evans KL, et al. Quantification of intracompartmental pressure and volume under plaster casts. J Bone Joint Surg Am 1981;63(3):449–53.

32. Coccolini F, Improta M, Picetti E, et al. Timing of surgical intervention for compartment syndrome in different body region: systematic review of the literature. World J Emerg Surg 2020;15(1):60.

33. Heckman MM, Whitesides TE Jr, Grewe SR, et al. Histologic determination of the ischemic threshold of muscle in the canine compartment syndrome model. J Orthop Trauma 1993;7(3):199–210.

34. Labbe R, Lindsay T, Walker PM. The extent and distribution of skeletal muscle necrosis after graded periods of complete ischemia. J Vasc Surg 1987;6(2):152–7.

35. Finkelstein JA, Hunter GA, Hu RW. Lower limb compartment syndrome: course after delayed fasciotomy. J Trauma 1996;40(3):342–4.

36. Ritenour AE, Dorlac WC, Fang R, et al. Complications after fasciotomy revision and delayed compartment release in combat patients. J Trauma 2008;64(2 Suppl):S153–61 [discussion S152–61].

37. Reis ND, Michaelson M. Crush injury to the lower limbs. Treatment of the local injury. J Bone Joint Surg Am 1986;68(3):414–8.

38. Troutman DA, Dougherty MJ, Spivack AI, et al. Updated strategies to treat acute arterial complications associated with total knee and hip arthroplasty. J Vasc Surg 2013;58(4):1037–42.

39. Calligaro KD, Dougherty MJ, Ryan S, et al. Acute arterial complications associated with total hip and knee arthroplasty. J Vasc Surg 2003;38(6):1170–7.

40. Lachiewicz PF, Latimer HA. Rhabdomyolysis following total hip arthroplasty. J Bone Joint Surg Br 1991;73(4):576–9.

41. Hanandeh A, Shamia AA, Ramcharan MM. Sciatic nerve injury secondary to a gluteal compartment syndrome. Cureus 2020;12(7):e9012.

42. Elkbuli A, Sanchez C, Hai S, et al. Gluteal compartment syndrome following alcohol intoxication: case report and literature review. Ann Med Surg 2019; 44:98–101.

43. Tarlow SD, Achterman CA, Hayhurst J, et al. Acute compartment syndrome in the thigh complicating fracture of the femur. A report of three cases. J Bone Joint Surg Am 1986;68(9):1439–43.

44. Verwiebe EG, Kanlic EM, Saller J, et al. Thigh compartment syndrome, presentation and complications. Bosn J Basic Med Sci 2009;9(Suppl 1): S28–33.

45. Mubarak SJ, Owen CA. Double-incision fasciotomy of the leg for decompression in compartment syndromes. J Bone Joint Surg Am 1977;59(2):184–7.

46. Bowyer MW. Lower extremity fasciotomy: indications and technique. Curr Trauma Rep 2015;1(1):35–44.

47. Shaath M, Sukeik M, Mortada S, et al. Compartment syndrome following total knee replacement: a case report and literature review. World J Orthop 2016;7(9):618–22.

48. Smith JW, Pellicci PM, Sharrock N, et al. Complications after total hip replacement. The contralateral limb. J Bone Joint Surg Am 1989;71(4):528.

49. Vegari DN, Rangavajjula AV, Diiorio TM, et al. Fasciotomy following total knee arthroplasty: beware of terrible outcome. J Arthroplasty 2014;29(2):355–9.

Necrotizing Soft-Tissue Infections After Hip Arthroplasty

Travis B. Eason, MD, Christopher T. Cosgrove, MD,
William M. Mihalko, MD, PhD*

KEYWORDS

- Necrotizing infection • Fasciitis • Hip arthroplasty

KEY POINTS

- Necrotizing soft-tissue infection is a rare complication of hip arthroplasty that is seldom discussed in literature.
- There needs to be a high index of suspicion for potential necrotizing soft-tissue infection in patients with periprosthetic hip infections and toxic condition.
- Expeditious diagnosis and treatment with surgical debridement and intravenous antibiotics are vital in reducing patient mortality.
- Despite advances in medical technology, necrotizing soft-tissue infections still result in high mortality rates.

INTRODUCTION

Necrotizing soft-tissue infections (NSTIs) are severe, rapidly spreading, life-threatening infections that can present as periprosthetic joint infections. This orthopedic emergency requires a high degree of suspicion and early diagnosis and treatment. NTSIs are often rapidly progressive and frequently become fatal.

NSTIs can involve skin, subcutaneous fat, fascia, and muscle and can present differently based on the soft-tissue components involved. These infections most commonly begin with some sort of break in the skin to begin the infection. These can be minor scratches and abrasions, penetrating trauma, insect bites, or surgical incisions, but NSTI has been described to occur without an initial break in the skin. The most common and classic manifestation is necrotizing fasciitis, a necrotizing infection that rapidly spreads along fascial planes. Other manifestations of NSTIs include necrotizing cellulitis, adipositis, and necrotizing myositis. NSTI is ultimately a surgical diagnosis characterized by friability of tissues, dishwater exudate, and the absence of pus.[1] NSTI can occur in a variety of locations, most commonly in the extremities. The treatment of NSTI includes early diagnosis, surgical debridement, and intravenous antibiotics.

EPIDEMIOLOGY

NSTIs are overall a rare occurrence in North America, with approximately 0.4 cases per 100,000 people per year of group A Streptococcus (GAS) NSTI.[2] The incidence of all-cause NSTI is difficult to quantify due to variability of reporting practices but is thought to be between 0.4 and 5 cases per 100,000 people and is variable by region.[3,4] It is estimated that approximately 1000 cases occur per year in the United States.[5] The mortality of NSTI remains high at around 20%, with even increased mortality with comorbidities such as diabetes, human immunodeficiency virus (HIV), and older age.[4] Risk

---

Department of Orthopaedic Surgery & Biomedical Engineering, University of Tennessee-Campbell Clinic, 1211 Union Avenue, Suite 510, Memphis, TN 38104, USA
* Corresponding author.
E-mail address: wmihalko@campbellclinic.com

Orthop Clin N Am 53 (2022) 33–41
https://doi.org/10.1016/j.ocl.2021.08.001

factors of developing NSTI include diabetes mellitus, obesity, peripheral vascular disease, chronic renal disease, cancer, heart disease, lung disease, intravenous drug use, smoking, alcohol abuse, trauma, history of methicillin-resistant *Staphylococcus aureus* (MRSA) infection, HIV/AIDS, hepatitis, and exposure to invasive GAS infection.[6–14] Despite this, up to 40% of cases have no known risk factors.[6,7]

CLASSIFICATION

NSTIs can be classified as type I, polymicrobial, and type II, monomicrobial, infections.[15] Type I, polymicrobial, infections involve aerobic and anaerobic organisms. These infections are most often seen in elderly individuals with comorbidities such as diabetes.[16] These infections often start from diabetic ulcers, hemorrhoids, rectal fissures, and colonic or gynecologic procedures. Breach of the infection around the gastrointestinal or genitourinary mucosal surfaces can lead to a rapidly progressive Fournier gangrene in the perineum. Type I infections classically present with gas in the tissue, which can be difficult to distinguish from classic gas gangrene caused by clostridial organisms. Polymicrobial infections usually present in elderly patients or patients with multiple medical comorbidities. There are alternate presentations of NSTIs, such as progressive bacterial synergistic gangrene, which can be a more indolent presentation of a skin infection with ulceration that can become rapidly progressive.

Type II infections are caused by a single bacterial organism. Monomicrobial infections are commonly caused by GAS[17] but have been documented with MRSA, *Clostridium* spp., as well as other species. Monomicrobial infections are more likely to occur in younger patients without risk factors.

Some have proposed expanding the classification to include type III infections, which include aquatic infections such as *Vibrio vulnificans* and *Aeromonas hydrophila*. Type IV infections are fungal infections (*Candida* spp.), which occur almost exclusively in immunocompromised patients.[18]

DIAGNOSIS

Early recognition and diagnosis of NSTIs are key in successful treatment.[8] Many patients who present with necrotizing fasciitis or other NSTI do not initially show hard signs such as skin changes (bullae, necrosis, ecchymosis) and toxic condition.[19] Many cases are initially underdiagnosed as cellulitis, as most cases present with swelling,

erythema, and pain, without external symptoms.[20] In the case of a soft-tissue infection around a prosthetic joint, the prosthesis is likely to be involved. In the case of a fulminant periprosthetic joint infection, one must be wary of the potential NSTI. There should be a high index of suspicion for a potential NSTI in patients with a toxic condition or multiorgan failure to prevent fatal progression.

LABORATORY EVALUATION

Laboratory evaluation has shown to be helpful in stratifying patients with higher risk of having an NSTI. The Laboratory Risk Indicator for Necrotizing Fasciitis (LRINEC) score was developed using multivariate regression to help predict the presence of an NSTI. The LRINEC scoring system uses C-reactive protein (CRP), white blood cell count, hemoglobin, sodium, creatinine, and glucose. This scoring system stratifies patients into low- ($\leq$5), intermediate- (6–7), and high-risk ($\geq$8) categories. The original publication showed high positive predictive value of and negative predictive value for scores greater than or equal to 6.[21] There have been multiple retrospective trials and a recent prospective trial that have attempted to validate the LRINEC score, but these have all shown poor correlation in differentiating cellulitis from NSTIs.[22,23] Despite its limitations, the LRINEC score remains a useful tool in the assessment of patients with the possibility of NSTI. Other series have also shown hypoalbuminemia and thrombocytopenia as predictors of mortality.[24] Diagnosticians must know the limitations of laboratory evaluation and ultimately use clinical acumen in diagnosis of this complex disease.

IMAGING STUDIES

Radiographic examination can be of assistance in diagnosis of NSTI. Early in the disease process, there may be little to no signs radiographically. When gas-producing organisms are present, gas can be seen dissecting fascial planes on plain radiographs. In the presence of a prosthetic joint, radiographs are vital in evaluating the current prosthesis for preoperative planning. Air entrapment after total hip arthroplasty is common and does not necessarily indicate the presence of an NSTI.[25]

Advanced imaging such as computed tomography (CT) and MRI can be helpful in diagnosis but should be used judiciously because they can delay the time to debridement. CT can be helpful in identifying signs of necrotizing fasciitis such as thickened fascia. It can also show areas of necrosis or abscess formation.[26] MRI is more sensitive, showing edema along fascial and muscular planes but often takes longer to obtain. When there are no skin manifestations, advanced imaging can show the location and extent of disease to help guide surgical approach. Advanced imaging should be reserved for stable patients, patients without focal signs of disease, and patients with an unclear diagnosis. For patients with clear signs of NSTI, surgical debridement should not be delayed. Ultimately, diagnosis of NSTI is confirmed with surgical debridement.

TREATMENT

The mainstay of management of NSTI is surgical debridement, with decompression of the soft-tissues and removal of necrotic tissue. Patients should initially be placed on broad spectrum antibiotics, which should be narrowed with availability of surgical cultures. Patients presenting with NSTIs are typically critically ill and require a multidisciplinary team. Surgeons from multiple specialties are often required (general surgery, orthopedic surgery, plastic surgery). These patients almost universally require intensive care unit admission with aggressive resuscitation and often intubation. Infectious disease specialists are often part of the team to help guide antibiotic treatment.

Surgical Treatment

It is recommended that the initial management with debridement of NSTI should be performed by the first surgeon to diagnose the necrotizing infection. Debridement should not be delayed, as studies have shown that debridement within 6 hours of presentation leads to a significantly lower mortality rate.[27] Early debridement is so vital in the survival of these patients that transfer to a higher level of care is not recommended until after the initial debridement unless a surgeon is not available at the evaluating institution.[28] For patients with a prosthetic joint, orthopedic surgery should be consulted early to assist with the initial debridement and guide surgical approach. Approach should be thoughtfully chosen to best decompress the infection, debride necrotic tissue, facilitate implant removal, and allow potential reconstructive procedures.

Surgical debridement should be conducted in a systematic fashion. The recommendation is to begin with debridement of the skin, working deep to subcutaneous tissues, fascia, muscle, and bone. All devitalized tissue should be removed, and involved fascial compartments should be released in a manner similar to fasciotomies for compartment syndrome. All devitalized tissues should be removed until margins of healthy tissue are created. It is imperative that all devitalized tissues are removed without regard for further reconstructive procedures to prevent progression of the infection and potential fatality. With extensive disease, dual incisions may be needed to adequately decompress and debride all sites of infection. Amputation is often required with significant progression of disease that makes the limb no longer salvageable. During the initial debridement, multiple intraoperative cultures should be obtained to help guide antibiotic therapy. Patients are generally left with their wounds open with moist gauze dressings or with negative pressure wound therapy.

In the case of involvement of the infection with a prosthetic joint, the implant should be removed.[29] Because of the emergent nature of NSTIs, the proper instrumentations and personnel for implant removal may not be available at the initial debridement. Proper resources should be arranged for repeat debridement to remove any implants to help clear the infection. Repeat debridement should be performed early, around 24 hours after initial debridement.[30] Debridement should be repeated every 24 to 48 hours until the infection is cleared. The patient can then undergo closure of the wounds and any reconstructive procedures such as flaps or skin grafting as needed. NSTI requires multiple visits to the operating room with average visits between 2 and 5 trips.[11,31–34] Because the aggressive nature of NSTI, a 2-stage revision of prosthetic joints should be implemented with initial implant removal and revision of the prosthesis once the infection has cleared.[35]

Antibiotics

Antibiotic therapy is essential in the treatment of NSTIs. As a patient is undergoing evaluation and preparation for the operating room, broad spectrum antibiotic therapy should be initiated and should not be held for surgical cultures. Blood cultures, well as intraoperative cultures should be obtained early. Because of the high likelihood of polymicrobial infection, antibiotic therapy with MRSA coverage as well as broad-spectrum agents against gram-negative organisms should be initiated.[36,37] In regimens that lack anaerobic coverage, metronidazole or clindamycin should be added.[38] Ultimately, local epidemiologic patterns should be considered when choosing initial empirical antibiotic coverage. Once surgical culture results are obtained, antibiotic coverage can be narrowed.

Patients with a periprosthetic joint infection are typically treated with 6 weeks of intravenous antibiotic therapy. Generally, a 2-week antibiotic holiday is given after the completion of the antibiotic treatment before joint aspiration and culture. With normalization of inflammatory labs and negative cultures, patients can undergo revision of the arthroplasty.

CASE REPORTS

There are very few reported cases of periprosthetic joint infection presenting as NSTI. We found 2 reported case studies of necrotizing fasciitis in hip arthroplasty in the literature.[39,40] We present 2 further examples of rare cases of patients with NSTIs around hip implants.

Case Report 1

A 61-year-old man with a medical history of hypertension, traumatic brain injury, epilepsy, alcohol abuse, chronic pancreatitis, and hepatitis B initially presented with a right displaced femoral neck fracture after a fall out of his wheelchair. He was treated with cemented hemiarthroplasty through a direct lateral approach (Fig. 1). A prophylactic cable was placed intraoperatively. His initial postoperative course was uncomplicated.

The patient returned to the emergency department approximately 1 month postoperatively. He was in septic shock with appearance of an NSTI tracking from his hip incision to his groin, abdomen, and perineum (Fig. 2A–C). He had dishwater-type drainage from his hip incision. His laboratory results on presentation

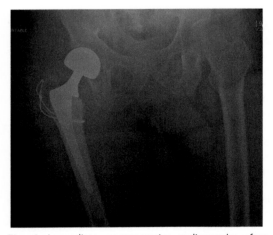

Fig. 1. Immediate postoperative radiographs after right hip hemiarthroplasty.

were white blood cell 42.3 k/mm^3, hemoglobin 7.5 g/dL, platelets 72 k/mm^3, sodium 128 mmol/L, international normalized ratio 4.59, creatine 5.3 mg/dL, C-reactive protein 201 ug/L, lactate 8.7 mmol/L, and glucose of 244 mmol/L.

The patient was placed on broad-spectrum antibiotics and brought to the operating room emergently for extensive debridement and irrigation by general surgery, orthopedic surgery, and urology. Intraoperative cultures were taken. His wounds were left open and dressed with a negative pressure dressing, and he was admitted to the intensive care unit where he underwent aggressive resuscitation and treatment of multiple organ dysfunction. The patient returned to the operating room a little more than 24 hours after the initial debridement for repeat debridement and explantation of his hip prosthesis (Fig. 3). Antibiotic beads containing vancomycin and tobramycin were left in the wound. Intraoperative cultures began growing methicillin-sensitive *Staphylococcus aureus* (MSSA). The next days he underwent multiple system organ failure, disseminated intravascular coagulopathy, and rapid medical decline. This patient had a total of 4 serial debridements before his illness proved to be fatal approximately 6 days after presentation.

Case Report 2

An 83-year-old man with no known history of major medical problems who had bilateral total hip arthroplasties done earlier initially presented with 2 weeks of increasing pain and swelling in his right lower extremity. He had not experienced a fever but complained of chills. He initially presented to an outside hospital where a workup included radiographs, CT of his right lower extremity, CT thorax, and basic laboratory workup. His vital signs at presentation were stable with a heart rate of 65 beats per minute, blood pressure of 101/51 mm Hg, respiratory rate of 12 breaths per minute, and temperature of 36.4° Celsius. His initial laboratory values were white blood cells 28.1 k/mm^3, hemoglobin 12.7 g/dL, sodium 130 mmol/L, glucose 117 mmol/L, and creatinine 1.25 mg/dL. Initial radiographs and CT of his right lower extremity showed extensive inflammation consistent with infection with subcutaneous and intramuscular gas tracking from the gluteus minimus and gluteus medius down the anterior compartment of the thigh (Figs. 4 and 5). CT of the thorax showed a small pulmonary embolism of the right lower lobe. He was subsequently transferred to a tertiary referral center for surgical treatment of

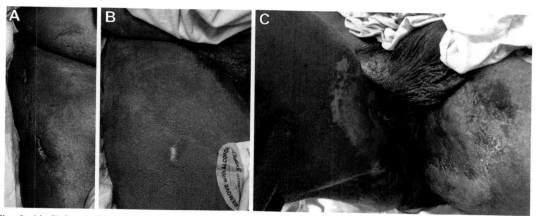

Fig. 2. (*A, B*) Surgical incision and skin changes on patient's presentation to the hospital. (*C*) Patient's perineum showed Fournier's gangrene at presentation.

his NSTI. A heparin drip for his pulmonary embolism and empirical intravenous antibiotics of vancomycin and cefepime were started.

The patient was brought to the operating room on an emergent basis for debridement of the NSTI. Dishwater-like fluid was found about the lateral thigh fascial planes. There were extensive areas of necrotic appearing fascia and muscle that were debrided. Intraoperatively, the orthopedic surgery team was consulted because of concerns about communication of

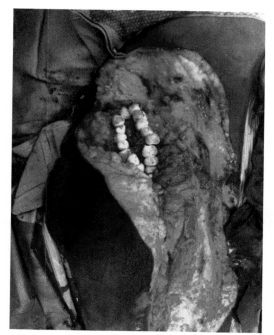

Fig. 3. Wound after the second surgical debridement and implant removal.

the infection with the patient's total hip arthroplasty prosthesis. The capsule, surrounding muscle, and fascia seemed necrotic in addition to extensive metallosis. The infection communicated with the total hip prosthesis with dishwater-like fluid found deep to the hip capsule. Intraoperative cultures were obtained. An extensive debridement was performed, removing all necrotic appearing tissue. The patient's wound was left open and dressed using a negative pressure wound therapy device and was transferred to the intensive care unit postoperatively.

Blood cultures grew gram-negative rods (*Morganella morganii*); intraoperative cultures grew gram-positive cocci (*Streptococcus anginosus*). No other organisms were isolated on surgical cultures. The patient's antibiotics were expanded to vancomycin and meropenem until sensitivities were obtained.

Approximately 36 hours after initial debridement, the patient returned to the operating room for debridement and explantation of his total hip prosthesis. The patient had a modular metal-on-metal total hip prosthesis that was implanted in 2004. The operative report and surgical records could not be obtained. The implants were all well fixed. There were still signs of infection with some dishwater-like fluids as well as signs of local tissue necrosis and metallosis from his metal-on-metal implant. His femoral prosthesis and acetabular cup were removed, preserving as much bone as possible. Thorough debridement and irrigation were performed. Absorbable antibiotic beads with vancomycin and tobramycin were placed into the femoral canal and the acetabulum. The wound was closed over a drain in layered fashion.

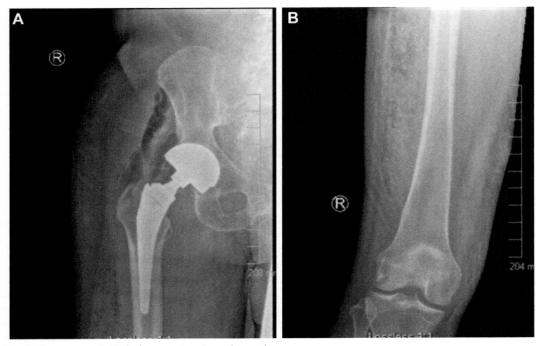

Fig. 4. Case report 2. Right lower extremity radiographs.

Postoperatively, the patient continued to improve clinically. Culture sensitivities were obtained, and antibiotic coverage was narrowed with guidance from the infectious disease team. Ultimately, the patient was placed on intravenous meropenem for a total of 6 weeks of treatment. He was transitioned from heparin to apixaban (Eliquis) for his pulmonary embolism. After an 8-day hospital stay, he was ultimately discharged home with intravenous antibiotics.

After completion of his antibiotic course, he was given a 2-week antibiotic holiday, and a hip aspirate was obtained. Aspirate results showed negative alpha-defensins, synovial fluid CRP less than .0.4, and no growth on aerobic and anaerobic cultures. The patient's serum labs of erythrocyte sedimentation rate and CRP had continued to normalize; CRP was 0.4 mg/dL and ESR had decreased to 40 mm/h. Once hip aspiration and laboratory values showed no further evidence of infection, we proceeded with the second stage of his hip revision: Girdlestone to a total hip arthroplasty (**Fig. 6**). Intraoperative cultures remained negative. The patient continues to show no signs of recurrence of infection and is doing well.

DISCUSSION

Periprosthetic joint infection of hip arthroplasty rarely presents as NSTI. When these do present, they require expeditious diagnosis and treatment with extensive debridement and often

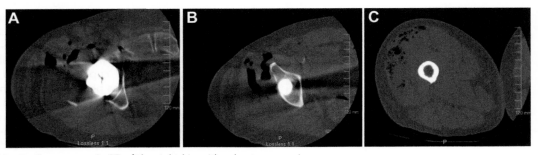

Fig. 5. Case report 2. CT of the right hip with subcutaneous air.

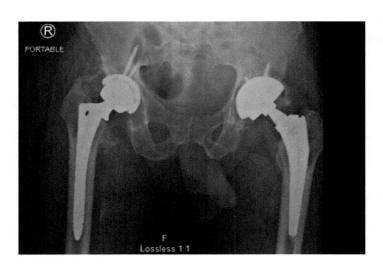

Fig. 6. Girdlestone to a total hip arthroplasty.

prove fatal. The first case of necrotizing fasciitis around hip arthroplasty was described by El-Karef and colleagues.[39] Their patient developed a superficial wound infection beginning 5 days after her surgery, which was initially treated with intravenous antibiotics. This infection progressed to a necrotic lesion, and the patient began to decompensate, necessitating surgical debridement. Cultures grew coagulase-negative Staphylococcus along with multiple other organisms. The patient responded well to debridement and plastic surgery coverage.

A different case reported by Sharma and colleagues described NSTI in a total hip that developed 10 days after surgery.[40] The patient had repeated debridement and removal of the prosthesis with placement of an antibiotic spacer. Cultures were polymicrobial, containing staphylococci, streptococci, and enterococci. Despite prolonged antibiotic treatment, a Girdlestone procedure was required because of persistent infection.

Our first case describes a patient who presented with a fulminant form of NSTI after a hip hemiarthroplasty. His infection was monomicrobial with MSSA but continued rapid progression of disease despite extensive debridement and antibiotic therapy. He quickly went into multiorgan failure and died from his disease despite what we would consider appropriate treatment. The presence of multiple risk factors—alcohol abuse, hepatitis, pancreatitis—likely contributed to his outcome.

The second case was likely type II, polymicrobial, infection with cultures growing Strep anginosus and M morganii. Strep anginosus is a Group C, beta-hemolytic streptococcus

organism that can be isolated in the pharynx, gastrointestinal system, and genitourinary tracts.[41] It is known for causing pyogenic infections with abscesses. In a retrospective review of 332 cases of Strep anginosus infections, Fazili and colleagues found that 72% of cases involved skin and soft-tissue and 9% involved bone.[42] They also noted that 70% of Strep anginosus infections were polymicrobial, most commonly with gram-negative anaerobes. M morganii (a gram-negative facultative anaerobe) was isolated in blood cultures but never in surgical cultures. It is presumed that the case was a polymicrobial infection, due to the isolation in blood cultures as well as the clinical presentation. M morganii is typically a communal organism residing in the human gastrointestinal tract. It is known to be involved in more indolent infections but can be involved in more aggressive polymicrobial infections as can be seen in this case.[43] In general, polymicrobial periprosthetic joint infections are rare and are associated with poor outcomes compared with monomicrobial periprosthetic joint infections.[44]

The initial imaging showed impressive presentation of air within the hip abductor musculature as well as the lateral thigh. During surgical debridement, the patient exhibited extensive myonecrosis along fascial planes consistent with necrotizing fasciitis. It is unclear whether the infection began as a periprosthetic joint infection or began as a more superficial infection and spread deep to the implant. With the absence of penetrating trauma or preceding skin infection, the former seems more likely. The patient presented with clear clinical signs of NSTI, with indications for emergent operative debridement. This patient was correctly treated promptly with emergent debridement. In our case, surgery was delayed by transfer to a tertiary care center, but this did not seem to negatively affect the outcome.

The patient had significant metal debris and necrotic appearing tissue around the total hip implant. The metal-on-metal hip arthroplasty may have been a contributing cause of this necrotic appearing tissue surrounding his hip. There is also some evidence that metal-on-metal hip arthroplasty has a slightly higher incidence of periprosthetic joint infection[45]; this may be due to Co-Cr particle-induced cytotoxicity and alterations to the host immune response.[46] Some have also hypothesized that development of pseudotumor, associated fluid collection, and necrotic tissue are ideal environments for the development of a hematogenous periprosthetic joint infection.[47]

SUMMARY

Periprosthetic hip infections can present as more aggressive NSTIs. These potentially deadly infections need to be treated with resuscitation, broad-spectrum intravenous antibiotic administration, and emergent surgical debridement. Of our 2 cases, one patient ultimately died from his disease, but we were successful in treating the other patient's infection with serial debridement, explantation of his retained implants, intravenous antibiotics, and reimplantation once the infection was cleared.

CRITICAL CARE POINTS

- Although rare, NSTIs can spread rapidly and have a high mortality rate.
- Early diagnosis and treatment are essential.
- Initial treatment is debridement and antibiotics.
- Removal of the total hip prosthesis may or may not be required.

DISCLOSURE

Dr W.M. Mihalko discloses payments from Aesculap/B.Braun (IP royalties, consultant, speaker), Stryker (research support), and Zimmer (consultant). Dr T.B. Eason has nothing to disclose.

REFERENCES

1. Bonne SI, Kadri SS. Evaluation and management of necrotizing soft tissue infections. Infect Dis Clin North Am 2017;31(3):497–511.
2. Nelson GE, Pondo T, Toews KA, et al. Epidemiology of invasive group a streptococcal infections in the United States, 2005-2012. Clin Infect Dis 2016;63(4):478–86.
3. Anaya DA, Dellinger EP. Necrotizing soft-tissue infection: diagnosis and management. Clin Infect Dis 2007;44(5):705–10.
4. Arif N, Yousfi S, Vinnard C. Deaths from necrotizing fasciitis in the United States, 2003-2013. Epidemiol Infect 2016;144(6):1338–44.
5. Sarani B, Strong M, Pascual J, et al. Necrotizing fasciitis: current concepts and review of the literature. J Am Coll Surg 2009;208(2):279–88.
6. Kalaivani V, Hiremath BV, Indumathi VA. Necrotising soft tissue infection-risk factors for mortality. J Clin Diagn Res 2013;7(8):1662–5.
7. Davies HD, Mcgeer A, Schwartz B, et al. Invasive group A streptococcal infections in Ontario, Canada. Ontario group A streptococcal study group. N Engl J Med 1996;335(8):547–54.
8. Goh T, Goh LG, Ang CH, et al. Early diagnosis of necrotizing fasciitis. Br J Surg 2014;101(1):e119–25.
9. Miller AT, Saadai P, Greenstein A, et al. Postprocedural necrotizing fasciitis: a 10-year retrospective review. Am Surg 2008;74(5):405–9.
10. Tan JH, Koh BT, Hong CC, et al. A comparison of necrotising fasciitis in diabetics and non-diabetics: a review of 127 patients. Bone Joint J 2016;98-b(11):1563–8.
11. Wong CH, Chang HC, Pasupathy S, et al. Necrotizing fasciitis: clinical presentation, microbiology, and determinants of mortality. J Bone Joint Surg Am 2003;85(8):1454–60.
12. Childers BJ, Potyondy LD, Nachreiner R, et al. Necrotizing fasciitis: a fourteen-year retrospective study of 163 consecutive patients. Am Surg 2002;68(2):109–16.
13. Glass GE, Sheil F, Ruston JC, et al. Necrotising soft tissue infection in a UK metropolitan population. Ann R Coll Surg Engl 2015;97(1):46–51.
14. Kong L, Cao J, Zhang Y, et al. Risk factors for periprosthetic joint infection following primary total hip or knee arthroplasty: a meta-analysis. Int Wound J 2017;14(3):529–36.
15. Giuliano A, Lewis F Jr, Hadley K, et al. Bacteriology of necrotizing fasciitis. Am J Surg 1977;134(1):52–7.
16. Stevens Dl, Bryant AE. Necrotizing soft-tissue infections. N Engl J Med 2017;377(23):2253–65.
17. Naseer U, Steinbakk M, Blystad H, et al. Epidemiology of invasive group a streptococcal infections in Norway 2010-2014: a retrospective cohort study. Eur J Clin Microbiol Infect Dis 2016;35(10):1639–48.

18. Morgan MS. Diagnosis and management of necrotising fasciitis: a multiparametric approach. J Hosp Infect 2010;75(4):249–57.

19. May AK. Skin and soft tissue infections. Surg Clin North Am 2009;89(2):403–20.

20. Stevens DI, Bisno AI, Chambers HF, et al. Practice guidelines for the diagnosis and management of skin and soft-tissue infections. Clin Infect Dis 2005;41(10):1373–406.

21. Wong CH, Khin LW, Heng KS, et al. The LRINEC (laboratory risk indicator for necrotizing fasciitis) score: a tool for distinguishing necrotizing fasciitis from other soft tissue infections. Crit Care Med 2004;32(7):1535–41.

22. Neeki MM, Dong F, Au C, et al. Evaluating the laboratory risk indicator to differentiate cellulitis from necrotizing fasciitis in the emergency department. West J Emerg Med 2017;18(4):684–9.

23. Hansen MB, Rasmussen LS, Svensson M, et al. Association between cytokine response, the LRINEC score and outcome in patients with necrotising soft tissue infection: a multicentre, prospective study. Sci Rep 2017;7:42179.

24. Tsai YH, Hsu RA, Huang KC, et al. Laboratory indicators for early detection and surgical treatment of vibrio necrotizing fasciitis. Clin Orthop Relat Res 2010;468(8):2230–7.

25. Smolle MA, Hörlesberger N, Musser E, et al. Air entrapment resembling necrotising fasciitis as a frequent incident following total hip arthroplasty. Sci Rep 2019;9(1):15766.

26. Carbonetti F, Cremona A, Carusi V, et al. The role of contrast enhanced computed tomography in the diagnosis of necrotizing fasciitis and comparison with the laboratory risk indicator for necrotizing fasciitis (LRINEC). Radiol Med 2016;121(2):106–21.

27. Nawijn F, Smeeing DP, Houwert Rm, et al. Time is of the essence when treating necrotizing soft tissue infections: a systematic review and meta-analysis. World J Emerg Surg 2020;15:4.

28. Lee A, May A, Obremskey WT. Necrotizing soft-tissue infections. J Am Acad Orthop Surg 2019;27(5):e199–206.

29. Parvizi J, Fassihi SC, Enayatollahi MA. Diagnosis of periprosthetic joint infection following hip and knee arthroplasty. Orthop Clin North Am 2016;47(3):505–15.

30. Okoye O, Talving P, Lam L, et al. Timing of redébridement after initial source control impacts survival in necrotizing soft tissue infection. Am Surg 2013;79(10):1081–5.

31. Elliott DC, Kufera JA, Myers RA. Necrotizing soft tissue infections. risk factors for mortality and strategies for management. Ann Surg 1996;224(5):672–83.

32. Misiakos Ep, Bagias G, Papadopoulos I, et al. Early diagnosis and surgical treatment for necrotizing fasciitis: a multicenter study. Front Surg 2017;4:5.

33. Angoules Ag, Kontakis G, Drakoulakis E, et al. Necrotising fasciitis of upper and lower limb: a systematic review. Injury 2007;38(suppl 5):s19–26.

34. Bulger EM, Maier RV, Sperry J, et al. A novel drug for treatment of necrotizing soft-tissue infections: a randomized clinical trial. JAMA Surg 2014;149(6):528–36.

35. Kapadia BH, Berg RA, Daley JA, et al. Periprosthetic joint infection. Lancet 2016;387(10016):386–94.

36. Ting NT, Della Valle CJ. Diagnosis of periprosthetic joint infection-an algorithm-based approach. J Arthroplasty 2017;32(7):2047–50.

37. Flurin L, Greenwood-Quaintance KE, Patel R. Microbiology of polymicrobial prosthetic joint infection. Diagn Microbiol Infect Dis 2019;94(3):255–9.

38. Zimbelman J, Palmer A, Todd J. Improved outcome of clindamycin compared with beta-lactam antibiotic treatment for invasive Streptococcus pyogenes infection. Pediatr Infect Dis J 1999;18(12):1096–100.

39. El-Karef E, Tiwari A, Aldam C. Necrotizing fasciitis: a rare complication of total hip replacement. J Arthroplasty 2000;15(2):238–40.

40. Sharma H, Kelly MP. Acute near-fatal necrotising fasciitis complicating a primary total hip replacement. J Bone Joint Surg Br 2007;89(7):959–60.

41. Giuliano S, Rubini G, Conte A, et al. Streptococcus anginosus group disseminated infection: case report and review of literature. Infec Med 2012;20(3):145–54.

42. Fazili T, Riddell S, Kiska D, et al. Streptococcus anginosus group bacterial infections. Am J Med Sci 2017;354(3):257–61.

43. Liu H, Zhu J, Hu Q, et al. Morganella morganii, a non-negligent opportunistic pathogen. Int J Infect Dis 2016;50:10–7.

44. Tan TL, Kheir M, Tan D, et al. Polymicrobial periprosthetic joint infections: outcome of treatment and identification of risk factors. J Bone Joint Surg Am 2016;98(24):2082–8.

45. Anwar HA, Aldam CH, Visuvanathan S, et al. The effect of metal ions in solution on bacterial growth compared with wear particles from hip replacements. J Bone Joint Surg Br 2007;89(12):1655–9.

46. Hosman A, Van Der Mei HC, Bulstra K, et al. Effects of metal-on-metal wear on the host immune system and infection in hip arthroplasty. Acta Orthopaedica 2010;81(5):526–34.

47. Grammatopoulos G, Munemoto M, Inagaki Y, et al. The diagnosis of infection in metal-on-metal hip arthroplasties. J Arthroplasty 2016;31(11):2569–73.

Trauma

Compartment Syndrome in High-Energy Tibial Plateau Fractures

Brian A. Schneiderman, MD*, Robert V. O'Toole, MD

KEYWORDS

- Acute compartment syndrome • Tibial plateau fracture • Complications • Fasciotomy

---

KEY POINTS

- Acute compartment syndrome is commonly associated with high-energy tibial plateau fractures.
- Numerous patient- and injury-specific factors can alert providers to those at higher risk of acute compartment syndrome.
- The rate of deep surgical site infection after open reduction internal fixation for tibial plateaus with compartment syndrome remains high (20%–25%).

INTRODUCTION/BACKGROUND

Acute compartment syndrome remains one of the few true orthopedic emergencies encountered with relative frequency by the practicing surgeon. It is particularly common in high-energy tibial plateau fractures, such as those seen in **Fig. 1**, with a rate of 15% to 27% in Schatzker IV-V-VI patterns and fracture-dislocation injuries.[1–4] This may be in part caused by the regional vascular anatomy that when injured may contribute to rising compartment pressures. With the popliteal artery tethered at the adductor hiatus proximally and trifurcation distally, arteries and arterioles have limited mobility and may be less tolerant to displacement during injury.[5]

Similar to all cases of acute compartment syndrome, delayed diagnosis in the setting of high-energy tibial plateau fractures carries significant implications and is the principle driver of poor outcomes.[6–8] If untreated, compartment syndrome can lead to functional deficits, loss of limb, and potentially life-threatening effects.[6,8,9] Delay in diagnosis and treatment leads to longer hospital stays and higher in-hospital costs, and medicolegal implications for treating physicians.[10,11] As such, surgeons treating high-energy tibial plateau injuries must be well equipped to monitor for acute compartment syndrome, and prepared to intervene in an emergent fashion when clinically indicated.

There are several important considerations when treating high-energy tibial plateau fractures in the setting of compartment syndrome. Surgical techniques must be thoughtful of the complex bony and soft tissue environment, which frequently requires fixation regional to or within the inevitable fasciotomy wounds. Despite ongoing study regarding surgical technique, timing of fasciotomy closure, and wound management, the risk of deep surgical site infection remains high and occurs in approximately 20% to 25% of cases.[12,13]

RISK FACTORS

Predictors for acute compartment syndrome in the setting of a tibial plateau fracture continue to be studied to hasten diagnosis and initiate

---

R. V. O'Toole is a paid consultant for Smith & Nephew, and Stryker; and receives stock options from Imagen, and receives royalties from Lincotek, unrelated to this study. B. A. Schneiderman has no conflicts of interest to report.
Department of Orthopaedics, R Adams Cowley Shock Trauma Center, University of Maryland School of Medicine, 22 South Greene Street, Baltimore, MD 21201, USA
* Corresponding author. 11406 Loma Linda Drive, Suite 226, Loma Linda, CA 92354.
E-mail address: schneidermanMD@gmail.com

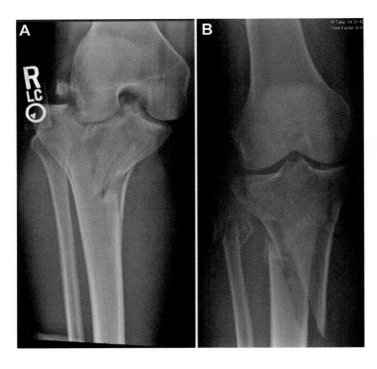

Fig. 1. Radiographic examples of high-energy tibial plateau injuries. (A) Schatzker IV pattern. A split/depression injury to the medial tibial plateau, with intact lateral cortex. Also, it is classified as a "fracture-dislocation" injury. The femur follows the short fracture segment, leaving the intact lateral plateau and remaining tibia effectively dislocated. (B) Schatzker VI pattern. A tibial plateau fracture (in this case lateral) with metaphyseal-diaphyseal dissociation of the tibial shaft.

treatment. Several nonradiographic and radiographic predictors have been identified to alert clinicians to those at highest risk.

Nonradiographic Predictors
Demographics
In fractures of any portion of the tibia, younger patient age has consistently been associated with increased risk of compartment syndrome, with age of 12 to 29 years being the single strongest predictor in a 2015 analysis by McQueen and coworkers.[7,9,11,14] Increased muscle mass and thicker fascial tissues have been proposed as explanations for the influence of age on acute compartment syndrome development, but high-energy injury mechanisms more common in younger patient populations may also play a role.[9] Analyses isolated to tibial plateau injuries largely reproduce similar results to those of other parts of the tibia.[5,15,16]

Male sex has also commonly been associated with acute compartment syndrome, in the tibia overall and when isolated to the tibial plateau.[15,16] Male patients exhibited an 8.7 times greater risk of acute compartment syndrome after tibial plateau fracture in a 2020 analysis.[15]

High-energy mechanism
Acute compartment syndrome has commonly been reported in association with injuries to any part of the tibia caused by a high-energy mechanism, such as those involving a motorized vehicle or fall from a height.[7,14,17] When defined as any fall from height greater than ground level, a motor vehicle accident, a motorcycle collision, a snow sport–related accident, or equivalent, a high-energy mechanism was found to confer an odds ratio of 3.1 ($P = .01$) in a recent study isolated to tibial plateau injuries.[15]

Although commonly thought to be reflective of high-energy mechanisms, open tibial plateau injuries do not confer a higher risk of acute compartment syndrome. Consistent with other regions of the tibia, the presence of an open fracture has neither been found predictive of nor protective against acute compartment syndrome in tibial plateau fractures.[7,9,14,15]

Ballistic versus blunt mechanism
In a review of 938 ballistic fractures throughout the musculoskeletal system, tibial or fibular injuries were found to have a four-fold greater risk of acute compartment syndrome. This risk was even more significant in proximal tibia and fibular injuries, in comparison with tibial shaft or distal tibia ballistic fractures.[18] Contributing factors again point to the muscular envelope of the proximal leg and the nearby vasculature, in particular the proximal nutrient artery to the tibia.[18]

Staged treatment

Staged management, consisting of temporary external fixator application and delayed definitive fixation, has been advocated to restore osseous length and alignment in tibial plateau fractures, while allowing soft tissue rest in patients not amenable to an immediate open approach.[3,4] It has also been suggested that traction applied to the extremity through an external fixator could cause increased compartment pressures in these acute injuries.[4] However, this latter hypothesis was not reproduced in a study that examined compartment pressures before and after external fixation in lower extremity trauma patients. In 22 patients with a preoperative compartment pressure to diastolic pressure differential greater than 30 mm Hg, none exhibited sustained pressure increases after external fixation that indicated a need for fasciotomy.[19]

Stark and colleagues[4] argued that fracture-dislocation patterns were at greater risk of acute compartment syndrome after external fixator application than were Schatzker VI injuries. Although definitive conclusions regarding the role external fixation may play in compartment syndrome could not be made, continued vigilant monitoring after temporizing fixation is strongly encouraged.[4]

Radiographic Predictors
Schatzker grade/OTA

When isolated to high-energy injuries resulting in Schatzker VI or fracture-dislocation patterns, the incidence of acute compartment syndrome increases up to 27%, because these fractures are theoretically accompanied by more significant soft tissue disruption and the possibility of vascular insult.[4] Further analysis reported 9 of 17 (53%) fracture-dislocations and 9 of 50 (18%) Schatzker VI injuries to be complicated by acute compartment syndrome.[4] Although the relative influence each injury characteristic has on compartment syndrome development merits further review, several studies have identified Schatzker VI injuries as having a heightened risk.[5,15,16,20] A similar association has been found regarding OTA/AO classification, with OTA/AO 41-C types carrying up to a 5.5 times greater risk than OTA/AO 41-A injuries.[5,9,15]

Combined plateau/shaft

In a retrospective 2017 study of 269 tibial plateau injuries, a noncontinuous tibia fracture, defined as a separate fracture complex of the tibia separate from the tibial plateau injury,

was found to portend higher risk of acute compartment syndrome.[16] Marchand and colleagues[15] corroborated this effect recently in a 2020 retrospective study. The influence of segmental injuries seems unique to plateau injuries, because Allmon and colleagues[20] reported no association between segmental tibial shaft fractures and acute compartment syndrome.

Fibular fracture

Concomitant fibular fracture in a tibial plateau injury has been demonstrated as a significant predictor for acute compartment syndrome, with an odds ratio of 2.39 to 8.14.[15,20] This effect has not been found in tibial shaft fractures or when all tibia fractures were examined.[14,20]

Fracture length

Fracture length, as determined by Allmon and colleagues,[20] was found to indicate increased likelihood of acute compartment syndrome development with odds ratio of 3.42. When examining all tibia fractures, the odds of acute compartment syndrome rose by 1.67 for each 10% increase in the fracture length to tibial length ratio. The authors proposed that an increasingly large fracture bed leads to greater blood loss and fracture hematoma formation, placing the surrounding tissue envelope at increased risk.[20]

Wahlquist classification

In a 2007 study of Schatzker IV tibial plateau injuries, Wahlquist and colleagues[21] proposed a subclassification describing the laterality of the fracture line as it exits into the joint. Type C injuries were those with fracture extension into the lateral plateau and labeled as fracture-dislocation injuries. Acute compartment syndrome was more likely in these patterns. Although not specifically classified in this manner, Stark and colleagues[4] described a similar effect in fracture-dislocation patterns. This was not supported by more recent publications that analyzed according to Wahlquist and colleagues, and it seems further review may be necessary to evaluate the effect of this subclassification system.[15,20]

Tibial widening/femoral displacement

In a study of 162 tibial plateau fractures, Ziran and Becher[5] described multiple radiographic measurements in relation to compartment syndrome risk. The tibial widening ratio, defined as the amount of tibial widening at its widest point in relation to the femoral condyle width, carried a 6.5 times greater risk of acute compartment syndrome when 5% to 10% wide.[5] Subsequent publications validate this finding as a valuable indicator.[15,16] In the same study, Ziran and Becher[5] also described the femoral displacement ratio as the offset distance between the anatomic femoral and tibial axes normalized to the width of the femoral condyles. Displacement greater than 10% was found to be a predictor of acute compartment syndrome, a finding substantiated in a 2017 study from a different institution.[5,16] However, the significance of femoral displacement is not ubiquitously demonstrated, with the largest published series on compartment syndrome risk factors in tibial plateau fractures failing to find an association.[15]

Evaluating Risk with Multiple Predictors

An analysis of 513 tibial plateau fractures by Marchand and colleagues[15] demonstrated that patients with more than one risk factor carry progressive increased risk of acute compartment syndrome. Factors evaluated included:

- Male gender
- Combined plateau-shaft fractures
- Schatzker VI fractures
- High-energy mechanism (defined as any fall from height greater than ground level, a motor vehicle accident, a motorcycle collision, a snow sport–related accident, or equivalent)
- Presence of fibular fracture

In the presence of three factors, the authors reported a 20% risk of acute compartment syndrome, which increased to 27% with four factors present. Although acute compartment syndrome can occur in any tibial plateau fracture, these findings serve to heighten clinician awareness and suspicion in the presence of high-risk patients, injuries, and patterns.

SURGICAL TREATMENT

High-energy tibial plateau fractures are typically managed operatively, with nonoperative treatment reserved for patients medically unable to tolerate surgical intervention. Traditional goals of treatment of tibial plateau fixation include anatomic reduction of the articular surface, and restoration of limb alignment, joint stability, and condylar width. These are challenging to accomplish in high-energy injuries that commonly present with significant displacement, comminution, and depressed articular fragments. Although Barei and colleagues[22] identified articular reduction quality (≤2-mm step or

gap) as the driving factor for outcomes in bicondylar tibial plateau fractures, this result is difficult to achieve and only accomplished in 55% of patients. Ultimately when anatomic articular reduction is not possible without significant soft tissue insult, emphasis should be placed on restoration of joint stability and limb alignment.

Soft tissue management holds even greater consequence for high-energy tibial plateau fractures with associated acute compartment syndrome, because the risk of deep infection in this setting is significant. A 2017 analysis demonstrated acute compartment syndrome to be the highest risk factor for infection risk in these injuries. Fracture classification alone did not predict surgical site infection when controlled for the presence of compartment syndrome. In the same study, deep infection rate for operatively treated tibial plateau injuries with acute compartment syndrome was 23%, in comparison with 8% for those without compartment syndrome.[12] The largest known cohort, consisting of 729 operatively treated tibial plateau fractures with fasciotomy wounds, found the overall risk of surgical site infection to be 19.6%.[13] Similarly, a 2020 analysis of 2106 tibial plateau injuries demonstrated compartment syndrome to carry a nine-fold greater risk of deep infection.[23]

Because acute surgical treatment in this clinical scenario is necessarily driven by the need for compartment release and decompression, surgical tactics focus on limiting infection risk in the presence of open fasciotomy wounds. Staged management, consisting of temporary external fixation, provides several advantages. It allows for the reconstitution of osseous length and alignment, while stabilizing the tenuous bony and soft tissue environment. Fasciotomy wounds are more accessible, facilitating monitoring and care. Soft tissues may rest, as clinicians continue wound management and plan for definitive fixation following the acute period.

Modifications in fasciotomy techniques and postsurgical care aim at decreasing infection risk and improving the healing environment for soft tissue and bone. Dual-incision fasciotomy has been the traditional treatment of choice for acute compartment syndrome, allowing surgeons optimal exposure for compartment evaluation and release.[24] A single-incision technique has been repopularized with proposed benefits including decreased soft tissue insult, improved blood supply to bone, and enhanced cosmesis, relative to the dual-incision approach.[25] Comparative analyses of the two techniques are limited, even more so when restricted to the context of tibial plateau fractures.

Bible and colleagues[26] retrospectively investigated the topic in 175 tibial plateau or shaft fractures with concurrent compartment syndrome treated with either intramedullary or plate fixation. Of the 81 patients treated with plate fixation, the single-incision group carried a 25.4% rate of infection, similar to a 22.7% in the dual incision group ($P = 1.000$). No significant difference was found regarding nonunion or need for skin graft coverage between groups. Of note, the plate fixation group included 27 fractures of the tibial shaft; however, the analysis remains the most applicable examination of single- versus dual-incision fasciotomies for compartment syndrome in tibial plateau fractures.[26] Decisions regarding single or dual fasciotomy technique should be based on surgeon preference and experience.

When treating compartment syndrome in the presence of a tibial plateau fracture, fasciotomy incisions must be planned carefully to permit definitive fixation. If made longitudinally 1 to 2 cm anterior to the fibula, a lateral fasciotomy incision can be extended proximally over Gerdy tubercle and into a conventional anterolateral approach to the knee at the time of definitive fixation (**Fig. 2A**).[27] However, when possible, some surgeons prefer definitive fixation through a separate incision, because of infection concerns of plating through a previously open wound. In this case, the lateral fasciotomy incision is planned more posterior than traditionally described and made directly adjacent to the fibula (**Fig. 2B**). This technique allows for a separate anterolateral knee exposure for definitive fixation of the tibial plateau, with a healthy skin bridge between incisions. The skin bridge is further optimized by minimizing overlap between incisions and by curving the proximal lateral fasciotomy incision posteriorly. In anticipation of continued swelling and subsequent deformation of the soft tissue envelope, each incision should be marked before making the lateral fasciotomy wound. In contrast, the medial fasciotomy incision is rarely modified, and simply extended proximally along the posterior border of the tibia when medial fixation is required (**Fig. 2C**).[27]

Following surgical decompression, fasciotomy wounds are managed with serial debridement, and other techniques to facilitate wound closure. Negative pressure wound therapy and a shoelace technique with vessel loops (ie, Jacob's ladder) may assist in wound contraction and achieving primary wound closure.[28–30] Wounds should be assessed for muscle viability and debrided as necessary every 48 to 72 hours. Closure may be considered safe when the wound bed is clean and no further muscle necrosis is appreciated.[27] However, surgeons should wait at least 3 days following fasciotomy to perform delayed primary closure, because earlier attempts have been associated with increased intramuscular pressure.[31] In the setting of dual-incision fasciotomies, the medial wound is typically closed first considering the proximity of the wound to underlying tibia and the minimal muscular coverage available.

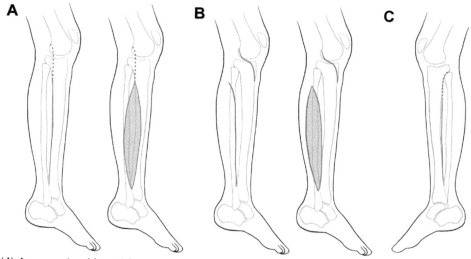

A   **B**   **C**

Fig. 2. (*A*) A conventional lateral fasciotomy incision and resultant wound may be extended proximally (*dashed line*) for lateral tibial plateau fixation. (*B*) The two-incision technique uses a more posteriorly based lateral fasciotomy incision to allow for a separate anterolateral approach to the tibial plateau when necessary. (*C*) A medial fasciotomy incision may be extended proximally (*dashed line*) when medial tibial plateau fixation is required.

Comparatively, the robust muscular envelope of the lateral leg is more amenable to skin grafting when primary closure cannot be achieved.

The timing of fasciotomy wound closure remains a subject of interest with theorized effects on surgical site infection rate. Previous work has demonstrated a 7% increase per day in odds of infection for each day to closure of fasciotomy wounds following decompression.[12] When considering fasciotomy closure in relationship to time of definitive fixation, prior analyses may not be sufficiently powered. However, a recently presented multicenter effort of 729 tibial plateau fractures with associated compartment syndrome found a statistically significant benefit of open reduction internal fixation at the time of fasciotomy closure (15.9% infection rate). Higher rates of deep infection occurred when fixation was performed before (20.6%) or after (21.6%) fasciotomy closure. These data represent a cohort 10 times larger than earlier examinations of the topic. Although the effect may be modest, there seems to be reduced risk of surgical site infection when definitive fixation is performed at time of fasciotomy closure.[13]

Fasciotomy wounds not amenable for delayed primary closure following debridement and soft tissue rest are candidates for split tissue skin grafting or flap coverage. Bible and colleagues[26] reported an approximately 40% rate for skin grafting in their cohort of 175 tibia fractures with compartment syndrome. This was similar to the rate of Ruffolo and colleagues,[32] in which 14 of 25 compartment syndrome patients required skin grafting. Of the 22 patients who underwent fasciotomies in Morris and colleagues,[33] nine required flap coverage, of which five developed deep infection. It was not reported how many of these injuries were open, and if traumatic wounds played a part in soft tissue management.[33] The need for some form of soft tissue transfer in tibia plateau fractures with compartment syndrome seems common, and further studies examining for a correlation between need for coverage and infection rate would be of value.

It should be noted that surgeons have several options when considering definitive tibial plateau fixation. Although open reduction internal fixation with bicolumnar plating for high-energy bicondylar injuries is a staple of operative management, circular or hybrid type external fixation, uniplanar external fixation, and percutaneous internal fixation may be indicated depending on patient and injury characteristics. Surgeons must be prepared to adapt preferred fixation strategies when mandated by the soft tissue environment and bony injury.

OUTCOMES AND OTHER COMPLICATIONS

In isolation, the evidence suggests that surgical treatment of high-energy tibial plateau fractures is associated with acceptable functional results. In 30 patients with a mean follow-up of 98 months, Weigel and Marsh[34] demonstrated satisfactory functional and patient-reported outcomes with a total range of motion arc 87% of the contralateral knee on average. A 2014 study of 74 patients reported more than 80% excellent and good results on multiple functional outcome measures with an average follow-up of 27 months.[35]

When evaluating for acute compartment syndrome, clinicians must weigh the lifelong complications following a missed diagnosis with the possibility of overtreatment and sequelae of fasciotomies. In a 2020 analysis of diaphyseal tibia injuries, patients with acute compartment syndrome that underwent fasciotomies had equivalent 5-year functional foot and ankle outcomes to patients without compartment syndrome. Compartment syndrome with fasciotomies correlated with decreased patient satisfaction, but equivalent patient-reported quality of life.[36] The totality of the literature is less conclusive, with variation reported in the rates of fracture nonunion, pain, neurologic symptoms, and undesirable cosmesis.[37,38]

Limited evidence is available regarding functional outcomes in the clinical setting of high-energy tibial plateau fractures and ipsilateral compartment syndrome. Barei and colleagues[22] showed no significant difference in functional outcomes between bicondylar plateau fractures with compartment syndrome and those without, although the study contained a small sample size. Treatment of these combined injuries focuses on complication prevention. Open regional wounds raise concerns for contamination and subsequent infection. Moreover, traumatic and iatrogenic devascularization of tissues may impede healing.

In general, nonunion for tibial plateau fractures is considered uncommon, occurring in less than 5% of fractures.[2,3,39] Although Ruffolo and colleagues[32] reported a 10.0% nonunion rate, this rate decreased to 4.3% with septic nonunions excluded. It has been proposed that in the setting of acute compartment syndrome, the traumatic and iatrogenic soft tissue insult may compromise fracture healing, leading to delayed union or nonunion. Barei and colleagues[2] reported 1 nonunion in 83 high-energy fracture patterns with ipsilateral compartment syndrome. In contrast Blair and colleagues[40] reported a 9% nonunion rate, albeit in a cohort of 23 patients. When controlled for smoking, no significant difference in nonunion was found with the control group of injuries without acute compartment syndrome. Small sample size is once again an issue for studies examining nonunion in the context of tibial plateau injuries with compartment syndrome. However, it seems tibial plateau fractures are not at significantly increased risk of nonunion in the presence of compartment syndrome, unlike tibial shaft fractures, which may be more susceptible.[40,41]

CLINICS CARE POINTS

- Known risk factors for the development of compartment syndrome include male gender, combined tibial plateau-shaft fracture, Schatzker VI classification, high-energy mechanism, and fibular fracture. Patients with more risk factors have increased risk of acute compartment syndrome development. The presence of four factors carried a 27% risk of acute compartment syndrome.[15]

- In the setting of a high-energy tibial plateau fracture complicated by acute compartment syndrome, the need for emergent four-compartment fasciotomies drives acute management, with subsequent staged treatment of the bony injury to follow.[28]

- Acute compartment syndrome is the most significant predictor of infection associated with surgical treatment of tibial plateau fractures, even more so than higher grade injury patterns. Overall infection rate in this clinical scenario is approximately 20% to 25%.[12,13,23]

- The choice of fasciotomy technique (single vs dual) has not been demonstrated to influence infection rate.[26]

- Fasciotomy wound closure at the time of definitive tibial plateau fixation is associated with a modest reduction in deep infection risk.[13]

SUMMARY

A high-energy tibial plateau fracture with ipsilateral acute compartment syndrome is a complex clinical scenario that demands specialized attention. Clinicians must be aware of the several risk factors that place patients at high risk for compartment syndrome development in these fractures. Expedient diagnosis and emergent surgical decompressive fasciotomies are paramount in preventing the negative sequelae of a delayed or missed diagnosis. When acute compartment syndrome is encountered in this setting, external fixation is typically performed for axially unstable patterns at the same time. Thoughtful and deliberate soft tissue management is required considering the eventual need for definitive fixation of the tibial plateau regional to fasciotomy wounds. Further understanding of nuanced aspects of management, such as timing of fasciotomy closure, type of coverage, mode of fixation, and postoperative care, is needed in the context of these concomitant injuries. Larger patient cohorts are necessary if more definitive claims are to be made.

REFERENCES

1. Firoozabadi R, Schneidkraut J, Beingessner D, et al. Hyperextension varus bicondylar tibial plateau fracture pattern: diagnosis and treatment strategies. J Orthop Trauma 2016;30(5):e152–7.
2. Barei DP, Nork SE, Mills WJ, et al. Complications associated with internal fixation of high-energy bicondylar tibial plateau fractures utilizing a two-incision technique. J Orthop Trauma 2004;18(10):649–57.
3. Egol KA, Tejwani NC, Capla EL, et al. Staged management of high-energy proximal tibia fractures (OTA types 41): the results of a prospective, standardized protocol. J Orthop Trauma 2005;19(7): 448–55. ; discussion 456.
4. Stark E, Stucken C, Trainer G, et al. Compartment syndrome in Schatzker type VI plateau fractures and medial condylar fracture-dislocations treated with temporary external fixation. J Orthop Trauma 2009;23(7):502–6.
5. Ziran BH, Becher SJ. Radiographic predictors of compartment syndrome in tibial plateau fractures. J Orthop Trauma 2013;27(11):612–5.
6. Finkelstein JA, Hunter GA, Hu RW. Lower limb compartment syndrome: course after delayed fasciotomy. J Trauma 1996;40(3):342–4.
7. McQueen MM, Duckworth AD, Aitken SA, et al. Predictors of compartment syndrome after tibial fracture. J Orthop Trauma 2015;29(10):451–5.
8. McQueen MM, Christie J, Court-Brown CM. Acute compartment syndrome in tibial diaphyseal fractures. J Bone Joint Surg Br 1996;78(1):95–8.
9. Beebe MJ, Auston DA, Quade JH, et al. OTA/AO classification is highly predictive of acute compartment syndrome after tibia fracture: a cohort of 2885 Fractures. J Orthop Trauma 2017;31(11):600–5.
10. Crespo AM, Manoli A 3rd, Konda SR, et al. Development of compartment syndrome negatively impacts length of stay and cost after tibia fracture. J Orthop Trauma 2015;29(7):312–5.
11. Shadgan B, Pereira G, Menon M, et al. Risk factors for acute compartment syndrome of the leg

associated with tibial diaphyseal fractures in adults. J Orthop Traumatol 2015;16(3):185–92.

12. Dubina AG, Paryavi E, Manson TT, et al. Surgical site infection in tibial plateau fractures with ipsilateral compartment syndrome. Injury 2017;48(2):495–500.

13. Dubina A, Morcos G, O'Hara N, et al. What is the appropriate time for ORIF of tibial plateau fractures with an ipsilateral compartment syndrome? A multicenter retrospective review. Paper presented at: Orthopaedic Trauma Association Annual Meeting; October 2, 2020, 2020; (Virtual).

14. Park S, Ahn J, Gee AO, et al. Compartment syndrome in tibial fractures. J Orthop Trauma 2009;23(7):514–8.

15. Marchand LS, Working ZM, Rane AA, et al. Compartment syndrome in tibial plateau fractures: do previously established predictors have external validity? J Orthop Trauma 2020;34(5):238–43.

16. Gamulin A, Lubbeke A, Belinga P, et al. Clinical and radiographic predictors of acute compartment syndrome in the treatment of tibial plateau fractures: a retrospective cohort study. BMC Musculoskelet Disord 2017;18(1):307.

17. McQueen MM, Gaston P, Court-Brown CM. Acute compartment syndrome. Who is at risk? J Bone Joint Surg Br 2000;82(2):200–3.

18. Meskey T, Hardcastle J, O'Toole RV. Are certain fractures at increased risk for compartment syndrome after civilian ballistic injury? J Trauma 2011;71(5):1385–9.

19. Egol KA, Bazzi J, McLaurin TM, et al. The effect of knee-spanning external fixation on compartment pressures in the leg. J Orthop Trauma 2008;22(10):680–5.

20. Allmon C, Greenwell P, Paryavi E, et al. Radiographic predictors of compartment syndrome occurring after tibial fracture. J Orthop Trauma 2016;30(7):387–91.

21. Wahlquist M, Iaguilli N, Ebraheim N, et al. Medial tibial plateau fractures: a new classification system. J Trauma 2007;63(6):1418–21.

22. Barei DP, Nork SE, Mills WJ, et al. Functional outcomes of severe bicondylar tibial plateau fractures treated with dual incisions and medial and lateral plates. J Bone Joint Surg Am 2006;88(8):1713–21.

23. Henkelmann R, Frosch KH, Mende M, et al. Risk factors for deep surgical site infection in patients with operatively treated tibial plateau fractures: a retrospective multicenter study. J Orthop Trauma 2020; 35(7):371–7.

24. Mubarak SJ, Owen CA. Double-incision fasciotomy of the leg for decompression in compartment syndromes. J Bone Joint Surg Am 1977;59(2):184–7.

25. Maheshwari R, Taitsman LA, Barei DP. Single-incision fasciotomy for compartmental syndrome of the leg in patients with diaphyseal tibial fractures. J Orthop Trauma 2008;22(10):723–30.

26. Bible JE, McClure DJ, Mir HR. Analysis of single-incision versus dual-incision fasciotomy for tibial

27. Crist BD, Della Rocca GJ, Stannard JP. Compartment syndrome surgical management techniques associated with tibial plateau fractures. J Knee Surg 2010;23(1):3–7.

28. Osborn CPM, Schmidt AH. Management of acute compartment syndrome. J Am Acad Orthop Surg 2020;28(3):e108–14.

29. Zannis J, Angobaldo J, Marks M, et al. Comparison of fasciotomy wound closures using traditional dressing changes and the vacuum-assisted closure device. Ann Plast Surg 2009;62(4):407–9.

30. Johnson LS, Chaar M, Ball CG, et al. Management of extremity fasciotomy sites prospective randomized evaluation of two techniques. Am J Surg 2018;216(4):736–9.

31. Wiger P, Tkaczuk P, Styf J. Secondary wound closure following fasciotomy for acute compartment syndrome increases intramuscular pressure. J Orthop Trauma 1998;12(2):117–21.

32. Ruffolo MR, Gettys FK, Montijo HE, et al. Complications of high-energy bicondylar tibial plateau fractures treated with dual plating through 2 incisions. J Orthop Trauma 2015;29(2):85–90.

33. Morris BJ, Unger RZ, Archer KR, et al. Risk factors of infection after ORIF of bicondylar tibial plateau fractures. J Orthop Trauma 2013;27(9):e196–200.

34. Weigel DP, Marsh JL. High-energy fractures of the tibial plateau. Knee function after longer follow-up. J Bone Joint Surg Am 2002;84(9):1541–51.

35. Yao Y, Lv H, Zan J, et al. Functional outcomes of bicondylar tibial plateau fractures treated with dual buttress plates and risk factors: a case series. Injury 2014;45(12):1980–4.

36. MacKenzie SA, Carter TH, MacDonald D, et al. Long-term outcomes of fasciotomy for acute compartment syndrome after a fracture of the tibial diaphysis. J Orthop Trauma 2020;34(10):512–7.

37. Fitzgerald AM, Gaston P, Wilson Y, et al. Long-term sequelae of fasciotomy wounds. Br J Plast Surg 2000;53(8):690–3.

38. Heemskerk J, Kitslaar P. Acute compartment syndrome of the lower leg: retrospective study on prevalence, technique, and outcome of fasciotomies. World J Surg 2003;27(6):744–7.

39. Berkson EM, Virkus WW. High-energy tibial plateau fractures. J Am Acad Orthop Surg 2006;14(1):20–31.

40. Blair JA, Stoops TK, Doarn MC, et al. Infection and nonunion after fasciotomy for compartment syndrome associated with tibia fractures: a matched cohort comparison. J Orthop Trauma 2016;30(7):392–6.

41. Reverte MM, Dimitriou R, Kanakaris NK, et al. What is the effect of compartment syndrome and fasciotomies on fracture healing in tibial fractures? Injury 2011;42(12):1402–7.

Pediatrics

Controversies in the Management of Unstable Slipped Capital Femoral Epiphysis

Shaunette Davey, DO[a,*], Tuesday Fisher, MD[b],
Tim Schrader, MD[a]

KEYWORDS

- Slipped capital femoral epiphysis • SCFE • Unstable SCFE • Pediatric hip disorders
- Avascular necrosis • Modified dunn osteotomy

KEY POINTS

- Slipped capital femoral epiphysis is the most common hip disorder in children.
- The primary treatment goal includes the prevention of slip progression by stabilizing the epiphysis while avoiding complications.
- There remains controversy about the optimal management of unstable slips as it relates to technique, timing, capsulotomy with rates of avascular necrosis up to 60% in the literature.

INTRODUCTION

First described by the French surgeon Ambroise Pare in the sixteenth century, slipped capital femoral epiphysis (SCFE) remains a disease that both intrigues and divides the orthopedic community.[1] SCFE is defined as anterior superior displacement of the metaphysis of the proximal femur whereas the epiphysis remains within the acetabulum. It is the most common hip disorder affecting the pediatric and adolescent populations, with a variable reported incidence of 0.71 to 10.8 per 100,000.[2,3] The incidence of SCFE in Polynesian, Black, and Hispanic children is 5.6, 3.94, and 2.53 times higher, respectively, when compared with Caucasian children.[3,4] SCFE more commonly affects boys with a male-to-female ratio of 1.5. The age of onset of SCFE is 12.7 to 13.5 years for boys and 11.2 to 12 years for girls.[4,5] There is also seasonal and geographic variability with higher incidence in the north and western parts of the United States than rates in the Midwest and South.

DIAGNOSIS

The diagnosis of SCFE is largely based on the physical examination supported by radiographic imaging. However, careful history also plays an important diagnostic role. Specifically, the duration of symptoms provides pertinent information as to the acuity or chronicity of the slip. A retrospective analysis of 82 unstable SCFEs found that greater than 85% of patients had symptoms before the onset of the slip, with an average duration of symptoms up to 6 weeks before SCFE.[6] Pain location is relevant as SCFE can also manifest as knee pain. The diagnosis can often be missed or delayed especially in patients who present with knee rather than hip pain and those who do not report severe pain. The history should also include changes in gait or weight-bearing status.

The classification system as described by Loder and colleagues is based on physeal stability to predict prognosis. A stable slip is defined as having the ability to bear weight with or

---

[a] Children's Healthcare of Atlanta, 5445 Meridian Mark Road, Suite 250, Atlanta, GA 30342, USA; [b] Department of Surgery, Uniformed Services University of the Health Sciences, Bethesda, *MD* 20814, USA
* Corresponding author.
E-mail address: sdavey14@gmail.com

Orthop Clin N Am 53 (2022) 51–56
https://doi.org/10.1016/j.ocl.2021.09.003

without crutches, whereas unstable slips are ones whereby walking is not possible even with crutch assistance.[7] The Loder classification has come under scrutiny in that it lacks mechanical implications for stability. Stability can be defined as whether the metaphysis moves in unison with the epiphysis. Unstable slips are present when there is independent movement between the metaphysis and epiphysis at the time of surgery.[8]

Physical examination findings suggestive of SCFE include limping, limited hip flexion, and internal rotation, and pain with internal rotation.[9,10] Drehmann's sign, which refers to abduction and external rotation of the hip with passive flexion, is a diagnostic finding. Bilateral lower extremity motion and rotational profiles should be documented and compared with identify motion restrictions that can occur in multiple planes.

Radiographic workup for SCFE includes anteroposterior (AP) pelvis and frog-leg lateral radiographs. Klein's line is the most widely known radiographic measure of SCFE. This is determined by a line drawn along the femoral neck that should intersect the epiphysis. Loss of this intersection correlates with a slip. However, early slips may show more subtle findings such as widening or irregularity of the physis, sharpening of the metaphyseal border of the femoral head, periosteal elevation, loss of anterior concavity to head–neck junction, and metaphyseal blanch sign of Steel which is a double density seen on AP radiographs due to the posterior slip of the epiphysis.[11] Fig. 1.

TREATMENT

The primary goal of treatment of SCFE is to stabilize the physis thereby preventing slip progression and avoiding complications such as chondrolysis and avascular necrosis. In situ screw fixation is the gold standard in the management of SCFE as it is a utilitarian technique that can be performed by all orthopedic surgeons. Despite its widespread use, the application and adjunctive procedures used with in situ screw fixation remain controversial. Utilization of this technique for surgical treatment of unstable slips, and current controversies, will be further discussed in this section.

In Situ Pinning

The widespread use of in situ fixation in SCFE is based on the work of Boyer and colleagues who reported on the satisfactory outcome of 121 patients followed for up to 47 years. In their study, patients with more severe slips fared better with in situ pinning than those in whom reduction was attempted.[12] This study highlighted the role of proximal femoral physeal remodeling after SCFE. The remodeling that occurs with time has also been supported in additional studies. Proponents of this theory believe that the residual deformity poses no clinically significant long-term sequelae and as such, in situ fixation is useful in the management of unstable slips.[13–15] In contrast, others argue that the potential deformity may be significant and initial management should involve more aggressive primary procedures.

The controversy surrounding the treatment of SCFE has been fostered by the paucity of literature regarding the outcome of in situ fixation for unstable slips. In a comparative study, the outcomes of stable versus unstable SCFE after in situ fixation were reported by Lang and colleagues who found 11.1% AVN of femoral head in unstable slips whereas a 1.2% incidence was found in stable slips.[16] This study evaluated 184 SCFEs, 9.8% of which were unstable; however, the mean follow time was only 3.2 months which may not have provided adequate follow-up time to obtain a true incidence of AVN for these unstable slips. Wenger and Bowmar provided a review of the literature which included their experience with unstable slips and recommended that in situ fixation alone may not be sufficient given the rates of AVN reported in these cases. They also noted residual cam deformity should also be considered as it can lead to premature arthritis from articular cartilage injury.[17]

The literature available leaves several unanswered questions regarding the necessity of reduction, timing of surgery, number of screws, and whether to perform capsulotomy.

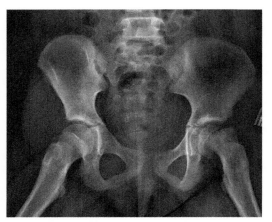

Fig. 1. Anteroposterior radiograph of the pelvis demonstrating SCFE of left hip.

Reduction Technique

Whether or not an intentional reduction should be performed at the time of in situ fixation is an area of controversy. Some authors argue that reduction has the potential to restore blood flow to the femoral head in the case of twisted or kinked vessels whereas others have concerns regarding the potential for iatrogenic injury to the retinacular vessels leading to the development of osteonecrosis.[18,19] Kitano and colleagues investigated risk factors for the development of AVN after SCFE and found that 7 of 21 unstable SCFE's developed AVN. The only factor that influenced AVN was closed reduction.[19] Interestingly, this was the case with deliberate reductions and "serendipitous reductions" (obtained with patient positioning). Based on these findings, they recommend not performing a reduction in unstable, acute slips. In contrast, Loder and Dietz provided recommendations in their 2012 systematic review of the literature which found that the best treatment of unstable SCFEs is gentle reduction, decompression, and internal fixation.[20] The senior author's practice is to assess physeal stability in the operating room and if unstable, a formal reduction using flexion, abduction, internal rotation followed by extension and adduction is performed, the joint is then reassessed and if deemed acceptable, we then proceed with in situ pinning.

Timing of Surgery

The optimal timing of reduction and operative stabilization in the management of unstable SCFE remains elusive. Unstable slips carry a significant risk of AVN with rates up to 60% in studies.[7,19,21,22] Timely reduction may lead to the restoration of blood flow to the femoral head thus decreasing the risk of AVN. In Loder's classic paper, the definition of "early" as it pertains to surgical timing, was not clearly defined.[7] A retrospective study by Kalogrianitis and colleagues sought to establish a recommended timing for reduction of unstable slips. They found that unstable slips are best stabilized within 24 hours of the slip, if possible, or to delay until 5–7 days to avoid the higher rate of AVN.[23] This study introduced the idea of an unsafe window for the timing of surgical management in unstable SCFE. This has been reviewed more recently in a multicenter study by Kohno and colleagues who evaluated 60 patients with an unstable SCFE treated with closed reduction and pinning or in situ pinning and found AVN developed in 16 of the 60 patients. The rate of AVN was significantly higher in patients with closed reduction and pinning who had surgical intervention between 24 hours and 7 days than those treated before or after this time (10 of 13 patients, $P = .002$).[24] There is inconsistency in the literature on how timing is reported. Some studies report time from presentation to the hospital while others report time from symptoms to surgical intervention. This heterogenicity makes it difficult to precisely draw conclusions on optimal surgical timing to avoid AVN or the concept of an "unsafe window."

Fixation with 1 Versus 2 Screws

One versus 2 screws in situ fixation has been another topic of debate in unstable slips. In his poll of North American surgeons, Sucato found near unanimous agreement that 2 screws are necessary for the management of unstable slips.[25] The rationale for 2 screw fixation has been stronger biomechanical construct with multiple points of fixation. This has been demonstrated in previous biomechanical models, whereby it has been found that 2 screws construct increases stiffness by 33% than a single screw fixation leading to a potential mechanical advantage.[26,27] This, however, may be technically difficult to achieve for some high-grade slips. In high-grade slips as the epiphysis displaces from the metaphysis, the safe zone to place a second screw across the physis narrows. This poses a risk for improperly placed screws and joint penetration. There are also concerns that multiple screws may increase the risk of osteonecrosis. This was reported by Tokmakova and colleagues who found a higher incidence of osteonecrosis in unstable slips treated with multiple pins.[22] Other authors have found no difference in the rate of osteonecrosis between single and multiple screw fixations. The senior author's preferred fixation is with one screw.

Capsulotomy

It has been theorized that hematoma and subsequent vascular compression could be a possible mechanism in the etiology of AVN in unstable SCFE.[28,29] There remains inadequate data in the literature to determine the best treatment method for or against capsulotomy. Herrera-Soto and colleagues reported the mean intracapsular pressure of unstable SCFEs in 13 patients during reduction and subsequent capsulotomy. The intracapsular pressure increased after manipulative reduction but dropped after capsulotomy and decompression.[30] In a meta-analysis reporting of pooled data of 17 articles with 302 unstable SCFE, Ibrahim and colleagues found no association between hip decompression and lower rates of AVN.[31] In contrast, Parsch and colleagues reported a 4.7% AVN rate in their study of operative management of 64 unstable SCFEs.[32] They attribute to this low rate of AVN to emergent timing of surgery, evacuation of the hematoma by performing capsulotomy, and gentle controlled reduction of the slip.

Vascular flow measurements before and after capsulotomy may provide a means to study the role of reduction and capsulotomy in femoral head perfusion. Schrader and colleagues reviewed 23 hips in which percutaneous intracapsular decompression was performed along with ICP monitoring.[33] (Fig. 2) At 2-year follow-up, there were no AVN cases in patients who had blood flow to the femoral head recorded on ICP monitoring at the time of the study. The best practice evidence has yet to be established as it pertains to capsulotomy. Further studies establishing the role of capsulotomy on femoral head perfusion with mid to long-term follow-up clinical studies are needed.

Modified Dunn

First described in 1964,[34] subcapital realignment osteotomy for SCFE has been modified and popularized over the past 2 decades by Ganz.[35] Advocates of the technique report correction of the head–neck offset and slip angle to near anatomic position due to the restoration of the proximal femoral anatomy.[36,37] However, the procedure is met with numerous potential complications, the most devastating of which is AVN. The most common complications reported in the literature after the modified Dunn procedure include, nonunion of the greater trochanteric osteotomy and implant failure.[37–39] In their report on 40 patients followed for 1 and 3-year minimum after modified Dunn procedure, Ziebarth and colleagues reported 0% osteonecrosis or chondrolysis.[37] Similar excellent outcomes from Ganz' institution in Bern have been reported by Tannast and colleagues, with a 2% AVN rate.[40] In a single surgeon retrospective study, Persinger and colleagues evaluated 31 consecutive hips with a mean follow-up of 27.9 months.[41] They reported an incidence of AVN of 6% after the modified Dunn procedure.

Despite such promising outcomes, these low rates of AVN after modified Dunn have not been replicated uniformly across other institutions. In a multicenter retrospective study, Sankar and colleagues evaluated 27 hips treated via modified Dunn technique and found a 27% rate of osteonecrosis with a relatively short follow-up mean of 22.3 months.[42] In a recent multicenter report of 21 hips followed for a mean of 40 months after modified Dunn, Masquijo and colleagues reported AVN rate of 47% in their series.[39] The modified Dunn is a technically demanding procedure with significant risks for devastating outcomes in the adolescent population. Surgeon and institution volume should be considered before performing this procedure. It is our recommendation that these cases are performed by a high-volume surgeon at tertiary referral centers.

We report the treatment algorithm in our institution used by the senior author for the urgent management of unstable slips. The surgical technique has been previously described by Schrader and colleagues with the use of intraoperative monitoring of perfusion pressure for in situ pinning.[33] Capsulotomy is routinely performed using a Cobb elevator. In situ pinning with one screw is our preference; however, a second screw may be necessary for high-grade slips due to persistent instability. We do not routinely perform arthroscopy or open procedures at the time of presentation of unstable SCFE. We believe that the stabilization of the slip is of utmost importance and that further treatment can be performed at a later time which may necessitate referral to a tertiary center for those not at these institutions. After in situ pinning, the patients are monitored at regular intervals with radiographs and clinical examination correlated with patient-reported symptoms. A modified Dunn is considered in patients with open physis, who report pain with deep flexion/impingement supported by clinical and radiographic findings. Magnetic resonance imaging (MRI) is obtained before surgical intervention. Other advanced imaging such as

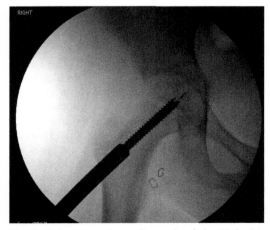

Fig. 2. Anteroposterior radiograph of the Right hip demonstrating in situ screw fixation with ICP probe into the epiphysis through a cannulated screw.

computed tomography (CT) scans and bone scintigraphy are not routinely used. The modified Dunn is performed as described by Ganz and colleagues.[35]

In summary, the urgent management of unstable SCFE is met with controversy as to the preferred operative technique for treatment. Further studies with mid–long-term follow-up are needed to best resolve this issue and to provide a clear treatment algorithm for Orthopedic surgeons.

DISCLAIMER

Some authors are employees of the U.S. federal government and the United States Army. The opinions or assertions contained herein are the private views of the authors and are not to be construed as official or reflecting the views of the Department of Defense or US government.

DISCLOSURE

The authors have nothing to disclose.

REFERENCES

1. Horworth B. History: a slipping of the capital femoral epiphysis. Clin Orthop Relat Res 1966;48: 11–32.
2. Loder RT. The demographics of slipped capital femoral epiphysis. An international multicenter study. Clin Orthop Relat Res 1996;322:8–27.
3. Lehmann CL, Arons RR, Loder RT, et al. The epidemiology of slipped capital femoral epiphysis: an update. J Pediatr Orthop 2006;26(3):286–90.
4. Loder RT, Skopelja EN. The epidemiology and demographics of slipped capital femoral epiphysis. ISRN Orthop 2011;2021:486512.
5. Novais EN, Millis MB. Slipped capital femoral epiphysis: prevalence, pathogenesis, and natural history. Clin Orthop Relat Res 2012;470:3432–8.
6. McPartland TG, Sankar WN, Kim YJ, et al. Patients with unstable slipped capital femoral epiphysis have antecedent symptoms. Clin Ortho Relat Res 2013;471:2132–6.
7. Loder RT, Richards S, Shapiro PS, et al. Acute slipped capital femoral epiphysis: the importance of physeal stability. J Bone Joint Surg Am 1993; 75(8):1134–40.
8. Fisher-Colbrie ME, Louer CR, Bomar JD, et al. Predicting epiphyseal stability of slipped capital femoral epiphysis with preoperative CT imaging. J Child Orthop 2020;14:68–75.
9. Peck K, Herrera-Soto J. Slipped capital femoral epiphysis: what's new? Orthop Clin North AM 2014;44:77–86.
10. Otani T, Kawaguchi Y, Marumo K. Diagnosis and treatment of slipped capital femoral epiphysis: recent trends to note. J Orthop Sci 2018;23(2): 220–8.
11. Georgiadis AG, Zaltz I. Slipped capital femoral epiphysis. How to evaluate with a review and update of treatment. Pediatr Clin North Am 2014; 61(6):1119–35.
12. Boyer DW, Mickelson MR, Ponseti IV. Slipped capital femoral epiphysis: long-term follow-up study of one hundred and twenty-one patients. J Bone Joint Surg Am 1981;63:85–95.
13. Carney BT, Weinstein SL, Noble J. Long-term follow-up of slipped capital femoral epiphysis. J Bone Joint Surg Am 1991;73:667–74.
14. Jones JR, Paterson DC, Hillier TM, et al. Remodelling after pinning for slipped capital femoral epiphysis. J Bone Joint Surg Br 1990;72(4):568–73.
15. Reinhardt M, Stauner K, Schuh A, et al. Slipped capital femoral epiphysis: long-term outcome and remodelling after in situ fixation. Hip Int 2016;26: 25–30.
16. Lang P, Panchal H, Delfosse EM, et al. The outcome of in-situ fixation of unstable slipped capital femoral epiphysis. J Pediatr Orthop B 2019;28: 452–7.
17. Wegner DR, Bomar JD. Unstable, slipped capital femoral epiphysis: is there a role for in situ fixation? J Pediatr Orthop 2014;34:S11–7.
18. Rached E, Akkari M, Braga SR, et al. Slipped capital femoral epiphysis: reduction as a risk factor for avascular necrosis. J Pediatr Orthop B 2012;21(4):331.
19. Kitano T, Nakagawa K, Wada M, et al. Closed reduction of slipped capital femoral epiphysis: high-risk factor for avascular necrosis. J Pediatr Orthop B 2015;24(4):281–5.
20. Loder RT, Dietz F. What is the best evidence for the treatment of slipped capital femoral epiphysis? J Pediatr Orthop 2012;32:S158–65.
21. Sankar WN, McPartland TG, Millis MB, et al. The unstable slipped capital femoral epiphysis: risk factors for osteonecrosis. J Pediatr Orthop 2010;30: 544–8.
22. Tokmakova KP, Stanton RP, Mason DE, et al. Factors influencing the development of osteonecrosis in patients treated for slipped capital femoral epiphysis. J Bone Joint Surg Am 2003;85:798–801.
23. Kalogrianitis S, Tan CK, Kemp GJ, et al. Does unstable slipped capital femoral epiphysis require urgent stabilization? J Pediatr Orthop B 2007;16:6–9.
24. Kohno Y, Nakashima Y, Kitano T. Is the timing of surgery associated with avascular necrosis after unstable slipped capital femoral epiphysis? A multicenter study. J Orthop Sci 2017;112–5.
25. Sucato DJ. Approach to the hip for SCFE: the North American perspective. J Pediatr Orthop 2018;38:S5–12.

26. Karol LA, Doane RM, Cornicelli SF, et al. Single versus double screw fixation for treatment of slipped capital femoral epiphysis: a biomechanical analysis. J Pediatr Orthop 1992;12:741–5.

27. Schmitz MR, Farnsworth CL, Doan JD, et al. Biomechanical testing of unstable slipped capital femoral epiphysis screw fixation: worth the risk of a second screw? J Pediatr Orthop 2015;35:496–500.

28. Herrera-Soto JA, Vanderhave KL, Gordon E, et al. Bilateral unstable slipped capital femoral epiphysis: a look at risk factors. Orthopedics 2011;34:e121–6.

29. Zaltz I, Baca G, Clohisy JC. Unstable SCFE: review of treatment modalities and prevalence of osteonecrosis. Clin Orthop Relat Res 2013;471:2192–8.

30. Herrera-Soto JA, Duffy MF, Birnbaum MA. Increased intracapsular pressures after unstable slipped capital femoral epiphysis. J Pediatr Orthop 2008;28:723–8.

31. Ibrahim T, Mahmoud S, Riaz M, et al. Hip decompression of unstable slipped capital femoral epiphysis: a systematic review and meta-analysis. J Child Orthop 2015;9:113–20.

32. Parsch K, Weller S, Parsh D. Open reduction and smooth kirschner wire fixation for unstable slipped capital femoral epiphysis. J Pediatr Orthop 2009; 29:1–8.

33. Schrader T, Jones CR, Kaufman AM, et al. Intraoperative monitoring of epiphyseal perfusion in slipped capital femoral epiphysis. J Bone Joint Surg Am 2016;98:1030–40.

34. Dunn DM. The treatment of adolescent slipping of the upper femoral epiphysis. J Bone Joint Surg Am 1964;46:621–9.

35. Ganz R, Gill TJ, Ganz K, et al. Surgical dislocation of the adult hip a technique with full access to the femoral head and acetabulum without risk of avascular necrosis. J Bone Joint Surg Br 2001;83:1119–24.

36. Upsani VV, Matheney TH, Spencer SA, et al. Complications after modified dunn osteotomy for the treatment of adolescent slipped capital femoral epiphysis. J Pediatr Orthop 2014;34:661–7.

37. Ziebarth K, Zilkens C, Spencer S, et al. Capital realignment for moderate and severe SCFE using a modified Dunn procedure. Clin Orthop Relat Res 2009;467:704–16.

38. Slongo T, Kakaty D, Krause F, et al. Treatment of slipped capital femoral epiphysis with a modified Dunn procedure. J Bone Joint Surg Am 2010;92: 2898–908.

39. Masquijo JJ, Allende V, D'Elia M. Treatment of slipped capital femoral epiphysis with the modified dunn procedure: a multicenter study. J Pediatr Orthop 2019;39:71–5.

40. Tannast M, Jost LM, Lerch TD, et al. The modified Dunn procedure for slipped capital femoral epiphysis: the Bernese experience. J Child Orthop 2017; 11:138–46.

41. Persinger F, Davis RL, Samora WP, et al. Treatment of unstable slipped capital epiphysis via the modified dunn procedure. J Pediatr Orthop 2018;38:3–8.

42. Sankar WN, Vanderhave KL, Matheney T, et al. The modified Dunn procedure for unstable slipped capital femoral epiphysis. A multicenter perspective. J Bone Joint Surg Am 2013;95:585–91.

Hand and Wrist

Necrotizing Soft Tissue Infections of the Hand and Wrist

M. Lucius Pomerantz, MD[a,b,*]

KEYWORDS

- Necrotizing soft tissue infections • Necrotizing fasciitis • Surgical emergencies

---

KEY POINTS

- Necrotizing soft tissue infections (NSTIs) are a surgical emergency that must be promptly addressed.
- The adequate treatment of NSTIs require a multidisciplinary team.
- The diagnosis of NSTI can be delayed or missed by confounding physical examination findings, laboratory test results, and imaging.
- NSTIs involving the upper extremity can be treated with amputation, but outcomes are not necessarily improved.

INTRODUCTION

Necrotizing fasciitis of the hand and wrist is a rare but extremely dangerous spectrum of infections that threaten the limb and life of the patient. It constitutes a true surgical emergency.[1–6] The term "necrotizing fasciitis" has been used due to the infection's fast spreading along fascial planes resulting in necrosis of the surrounding tissues. The term "necrotizing soft tissue infection" (NSTI) is another term often used for these infections and is a more generalized term that better covers the true spectrum of the disease. Prompt diagnosis and treatment are crucial to patient outcomes, and the care of these patients requires a multidisciplinary approach involving surgeons, infectious disease experts, critical care physicians, and many other supportive services.

Although rare, there is evidence of increasing incidence, and most of these cases affect the extremities. The upper extremity is less frequently involved than the lower extremity[3,6,7] with an estimated upper extremity involvement of greater than one-third of total extremity cases.[3,7] It is estimated that the upper extremities account for approximately 10% to 16% of total cases of NSTI.[6–8] Mortality rate of NSTI is estimated to be greater than 20% in extremity infections.[3,6,9–13]

NSTIs can have variable presentation from a hyperacute form to a more subacute form. Although the subacute form may progress over days to weeks, it is the hyperacute form that can progress in a matter of hours to life threatening. In these hyperacute cases, the extent of the infection is not realized until operating room debridement, as the skin manifestations have not yet had the time to declare themselves.

Because of the high mortality rate, prompt recognition and treatment is crucial. Unfortunately, the variable and often innocuous presenting symptoms make recognition difficult, and this often delays proper treatment. Early recognition of the signs and symptoms involve an awareness of vulnerable populations as well as having a high index of suspicion. Prompt surgical intervention is imperative with the expectation that multiple debridements will be required. In addition, a multidisciplinary medical approach

---

[a] Synergy Orthopedic Specialists, Inc., 955 Lane Ave, #200, Chula Vista, CA 91914, USA; [b] Orthopedic Surgery, University of California San Diego, San Diego, CA, USA

* Lane Avenue, #200, Chula Vista, CA 91914.

E-mail address: LPomerantz@SynergySMG.com

is necessary to optimize outcomes. This review article attempts to address recognition, pathophysiology, and treatment of this dangerous disorder with an emphasis on the upper extremity.

RECOGNITION/DIAGNOSIS

The initiation of prompt treatment starts with recognition of the problem. Unfortunately, the early recognition can be difficult, and it is often the difference in survival of the patient.[5,6,8,14,15] The most important findings lie in history and examination for early clinical recognition, but an understanding of the patients who are more susceptible can aid in making the diagnosis. Laboratory values and imaging are helpful in diagnosis, but surgical intervention should not be delayed if clinical suspicion of NSTI exists. The following section reviews the factors that can help make the diagnosis of NSTI. For common pitfalls in the diagnosis of NSTI see **Table 1**.[16]

PATIENT POPULATION

Multiple studies have identified patient populations more at risk of developing NSTI, but many patients have no underlying medical risks. One such risk is there may be a history of local trauma. However, the history of trauma may be remote or minor. Skin breaks in the form of chronic wounds, surgical wounds, or intravenous/intramuscular drug abuse are more obvious mechanisms.[3] Patients who abuse drugs are more susceptible to have these extremity infections[2,3,17–19] as well. If they inject the drugs then there will be skin breaks and poor sanitation. However, drug abuse contributes to a myriad of factors such as poor nutrition, altered mental status delaying recognition, and the direct effects of the drugs on the body that blunt immune response.[20] Diabetics are also at increased risk of these infections.[2,3,6,8,10,17,21] Those with suppressed immune systems from other factors such as human immunodeficiency virus[10,18] or other significant comorbidities such as increased age, peripheral vascular disease, cancer, renal disease, liver disease, and alcoholism are more susceptible.[3,6,8,13,21,22] The research specifically to upper extremity NSTI is very limited to small case studies, but it would seem that risk factors for upper extremity NSTI are similar as to what has already been described for NSTIs in general.[9–13]

Another patient factor in recognition is to be aware of any prior treatments; this includes the initiation of oral antibiotics by an outside physician, as this may alter the disease trajectory by lowering the bacterial burden initially. Some investigators have also discussed the use of nonsteroidal antiinflammatory drugs possibly worsening the course of NSTI either through masking signs and symptoms, by actual inhibition of the immune system, and/or augment factors that contribute to septic shock[4,16] although research to these points is limited.

SIGNS AND SYMPTOMS
Local Appearance

Initially, the findings may be subtle. There may be edema, warmth, or erythema, but the skin may look normal.[3,6,8] Initially, it may be hard to

Table 1	
Common pitfalls in diagnosis of necrotizing soft tissue infections	
Pitfall	**Explanation**
Absence of fever	NSAID use or *Clostridium sordellii* infection
Absence of cutaneous manifestations	Infections arising in deeper tissues (without obvious portal of entry) often do not have cutaneous manifestations until late in the course of the disease
Attributing severe pain to injury or procedure	NSTI is often accompanied by severe pain. However, pain can be erroneously attributed to an injury or recent surgery. With disproportionate pain, NSTI should be considered. Conversely, pain may be absent if there has been use of NSAIDs or there is diabetic neuropathy.
Nonspecific imaging tests	Often, even with more advanced imaging, findings can be confounding.
Attributing systemic manifestations to other causes	Nausea, vomiting, and diarrhea may be early manifestations of toxemia from group A streptococcal infection but may be attributed to food poisoning or other gastrointestinal illness.

Adapted from Table 2 of Stevens DL, Bryant AE. Necrotizing Soft-Tissue Infections. N Engl J Med. 2017;377(23):2253-65.

Empiric Treatment			
Vancomycin + Piperacillin/Tazobactam			
Cultures/Sensitivities			
Monomicrobial	**Antibiotic regimen**	**Polymicrobial**	**Continue Vancomycin + Piperacillin/Tazobactam**
Streptococcus pyogenes	Penicillin + Clindamycin		
Clostridial	Penicillin + Clindamycin		
Vibrio vulnificus	Doxycycline + Ceftazidime		
Aeromonas hydrophila	Doxycycline + Ciprofloxacin		

Fig. 1. Antibiotic Treatment for NSTIs. (*Data from* Stevens DL, Bisno AL, Chambers HF, Dellinger EP, Goldstein EJ, Gorbach SL, et al. Practice guidelines for the diagnosis and management of skin and soft tissue infections: 2014 update by the Infectious Diseases Society of America. Clin Infect Dis. 2014;59(2):e10–52)

differentiate from less dangerous issues such as cellulitis or small abscess. An incongruity in appearance and symptoms should raise concern. Examples of concerning findings include pain that is hard to localize, extends beyond the apparent involved area, or is disproportionate to the appearance of the tissues.[3,6] These are important findings that differentiate early stage NSTI from less dangerous disease.

It is after the initial stage that serous blisters and bullae can form (**Fig. 1**). As the disease process advances, these become hemorrhagic. It is also in the later stages that the more obvious changes consistent with NSTI occur, such as crepitus, skin anesthesia, skin duskiness, and overt skin necrosis, and gangrene. However, by the time these more obvious signs begin to present, significant morbidity to the patient has already occurred and the patient will often be showing signs of sepsis, septic shock, and/or organ failure (**Table 2**).

A bedside cutdown is a described diagnostic tool for detecting early NSTI before proceeding with definitive surgery.[1,4,17,23] Under local anesthesia only (best without epinephrine to better assess bleeding), a 2 cm incision is made in the area of interest down to the deep fascia followed by gentle probing with a finger—hence being called the "finger test." Some investigators have advocated using a 1 cm incision and a blunt hemostat on the hands and wrists. Findings concerning for NSTI include "dishwater" fluid, lack of resistance to blunt dissection, and absence of bleeding tissue/thrombosis of subcutaneous vessels.[4,21,22] The incision also provides an opportunity to obtain tissue for biopsy (rapid frozen-section) and culture with Gram stain.[1] However, the personal preference of this author is that if clinical suspicion is high enough to perform this test then doing a formal surgery in the operative arena is the best course of action.

GENERAL APPEARANCE AND SYSTEMIC SIGNS

Initially, the patient may seem completely normal. There will be normal mental processes and a benign generalized appearance. It is as sepsis sets in that altered mental status and other evidence of shock and organ failure begin to be apparent. The transition to these findings

Table 2		
Clinical features of necrotizing soft tissue infections		
Stage 1 (Early)	**Stage 2 (Intermediate)**	**Stage 3 (Late)**
• Tenderness to palpation (extending beyond the apparent are of skin involvement and/or disproportionate to appearance) • Erythema • Swelling • Warm to Palpation	• Blister or bullae formation (serous) • Skin fluctance • Skin induration	• Hemorrhagic bullae • Skin anesthesia • Crepitus • Skin necrosis with dusky discoloration progressing to frank gangrene

Adapted from Table 1 of Wong CH, Wang YS. The diagnosis of necrotizing fasciitis. Curr Opin Infect Dis. 2005;18(2):101-6.

can be abrupt. Hemodynamic instability can often be the first real clue as to the seriousness of the infection.[22] However, systemic symptoms such as tachycardia, hypotension, altered mental status, and fevers are variably present.[3,6,16]

DIAGNOSTIC STUDIES

Laboratory Values

Obtaining laboratory test results is a crucial component to early recognition of NSTI and contribute to providing systemic care. It has been shown in many studies that patients with NSTI have altered laboratory values.[2,3,6,24,25] Laboratory test results add to evidence that systemic changes are occurring that one might not expect, given the clinical examination in the early stages of the disease.

The Laboratory Risk Indicator for Necrotizing Fasciitis (LRINEC) score, as published by Wong and colleagues[25] (Table 3), is the most cited

Table 3 Laboratory Risk Indicator for Necrotizing Fasciitis score	
Variable, Units	**Score**
C-reactive protein, mg/dL	
<15	0
≧15	4
Total white cell count, per mm^3	
<15	0
15–25	1
>25	2
Hemoglobin, g/dL	
>13.5	0
11–13.5	1
<11	2
Sodium, mEq/L	
≧135	0
<135	2
Creatinine, mg/dL	
≦1.6	0
>1.6	2
Glucose, mg/dL	
≦180	0
>180	1

Adapted from Table 2 of Wong CH, Khin LW, Heng KS, Tan KC, Low CO. The LRINEC (Laboratory Risk Indicator for Necrotizing Fasciitis) score: a tool for distinguishing necrotizing fasciitis from other soft tissue infections. Crit Care Med. 2004;32(7):1535-41.

laboratory score in aiding in the diagnosis of NSTI. The laboratory test results necessary are easily obtained from routine blood testing. The investigators of the initial study found positive predictive value (PPV) of 92% and negative predictive value (NPV) of 96% when the LRINEC score was greater than 6. Although the LRINEC scoring system has been criticized and should not be the only diagnostic criteria used,[4,14,26–28] it is valuable in assisting in recognition of NSTI and assigning risk stratification. Subsequent literature has found that the LRINEC score can be helpful for diagnosis.[26,27] The LRINEC score is better at ruling out NSTI[1,28] and also does not provide significant information on disease severity or outcome.[11,14,29] In addition, in a study specific to Vibrio NSTI, all 18 patients who died had an LRINEC score of less than 6,[30] and another study on Vibrio NSTI recommended lowering the threshold score to 2.[27] The lack of consensus on the LRINEC score or other attempts at establishing laboratory criteria for NSTI is a consequence of the broad spectrum of presentation, pathology, and patients affected by the disease.

Imaging

Imaging studies can provide valuable diagnostic information, but one should never delay surgical intervention in cases of clinical suspicion of NSTI to obtain imaging.

Radiographs are simple and quick to obtain and should be obtained on all suspected cases of upper extremity NSTI when possible. Early in the disease process they may be normal, but as the disease progresses there may be findings such as increased opacity and thickness of soft tissues. Later findings such as air in the subcutaneous tissues (Fig. 2) or tracking along fascial planes are highly concerning and characteristic of NSTI but often not present.[3,6]

Ultrasound is also a simple and quick modality and has better soft tissue detail and utility than radiograph. It can provide a significant amount of information such as hypoechoic fluid between subcutaneous tissues and muscle or may demonstrate gas adjacent to the fascia. Unfortunately, ultrasound is not always available and subject to error by the administrating practitioner. Ultrasound is the preferred imaging study by Leiblein and colleagues[29] due to its higher information potential and relatively good accessibility in emergency departments.

Computed tomography (CT) is very sensitive and specific to NSTI[31–33] with CT with contrast having improved specificity.[32] CT scans can show dermal thickening, fat stranding, soft

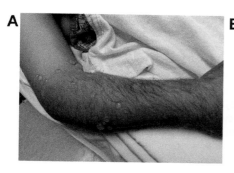

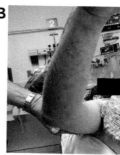

Fig. 2. Representative NSTI case of forearm. (*A*) Serous blistering/bullae on dorsal forearm. (*B*) Erythema and hemorrhagic changes on volar forearm.

tissue attenuation, and fluid and/or air in subfascial planes. CT is the most sensitive study for detecting gas within tissues, a highly specific finding, and it is a study that is relatively quick to perform and more accessible than MRI. McGillicuddy and colleagues[33] tried to establish a CT-based scoring system for NSTI. Based on their results, the presence of fascial gas had an odds ratio of 22.6 compared with nonnecrotizing infection and was weighted highest (**Table 4**). In their study, a score greater than 6 resulted in a sensitivity of 83%, specificity of 92%, PPV 63%, and NPV 86%. Although gas is the most diagnostic finding, it is not present in most cases.[31,33]

MRI is the best study for detailed images of soft tissues, but its utility for NSTI is debated. If examination, laboratory test results, and other more accessible imaging still have not provided sufficient evidence, MRI can be used to help distinguish NSTI from other infections—*if the patient is stable enough to undergo the study.* Contrast-enhanced MRI provides additional

detail. Pertinent findings distinguishing NSTI from other infection were that NSTI was more likely to have thickened abnormal fascial signal and low signal intensity in the deep fascia on fat-suppressed T2-weighted images, nonenhancing portions in the areas of abnormal signal intensity in the deep fascia, extensive involvement of the deep fascia, and involvement of 3 or more compartments in one extremity.[34] To reiterate, one should have caution using MRI, as it can delay prompt treatment.

Differential Diagnosis

The diagnosis of NSTI is often difficult due to varied presentation and nonspecific diagnostic tools. As referenced before, pitfalls in the diagnosis of NSTI are summarized in **Table 1**.

Cellulitis and abscesses have a very similar presentation to early NSTI. High index of suspicion should always be present when dealing with any infectionlike picture.

Open wounds, whether chronic or acute, can be the cause of air in the tissues and can confound an otherwise highly diagnostic finding to NSTI on imaging.

In addition, dermatologic conditions such as pyoderma gangrenosum can have an appearance of NSTI, as it progresses from a papule or nodule to painful ulcerated lesions with central necrosis.[35] However, in this condition there is no systemic involvement. Surgical debridement should be avoided in this condition, as it may exacerbate it.

Pathophysiology
Microbiology

Although several classification systems exist for NSTIs based on anatomic location or depth of infection, these do not contribute to clinical management or prognosis in any significant way.[4] However, classification systems based on the causative organism do guide clinical management. There are 4 general types of microbial

Table 4	
Computed tomography–based scoring system for necrotizing soft tissue infections	
Variable	**Points**
Fascial air	5
Muscle/fascial edema	4
Fluid tracking	3
Lymphadenopathy	2
Subcutaneous edema	1
Score >6 points was 86.3% sensitive and 91.5% specific (PPV 63.3%, NPV 85.5%)	

Adapted from Table 2 of McGillicuddy EA, Lischuk AW, Schuster KM, Kaplan LJ, Maung A, Lui FY, et al. Development of a computed tomography-based scoring system for necrotizing soft-tissue infections. J Trauma. 2011;70(4):894-9.

NSTIs (**Table 5**).[36] Giuliano and colleagues[37] were the first to describe the first 2, and most common, subtypes. For a summary of factors that may contribute to specific types of infections see **Table 6**.

(Below can be eliminated if the table is adequate)

Type 1 infections represent most of the cases and are polymicrobial. These compromise 70% to 80% of cases. Both aerobic and anaerobic organisms are present, often of bowel flora, and seem to behave in a synergistic way increasing morbidity. These infections tend to affect older patients with underlying comorbidities. They are usually slower spreading and affect the trunk and perineum. "Gas gangrene" from clostridial infections are a subtype of type 1 infections and can be associated with the injection of "black tar" heroin, but clostridial species are often endemic in the soil. These infections tend to be more rapidly progressive and with increased mortality,[2] even exceeding 50%.[4]

Type 2 infections involve a single organism. Most commonly it is Group A beta-hemolytic streptococci (GAS) or *Staphylococcus aureus*. These infections compromise 20% to 30% of NSTIs and can occur in any age group. They are seen in patients without any underlying medical conditions, but those with history of intravenous (IV) drug abuse, trauma, or surgery are those that classically fall into this subset. These infectious often involve the extremities. Toxic shock syndrome from the GAS often contribute the severe clinical nature of these infections.

Type 3 infections involve gram-negative marine bacteria. The most common of these is *Vibrio vulnificus*. It often involves an injury with exposure to marine environment, and patients involved often have moderate to severe liver disease.[27,30] This type of infection has an aggressive course, and mortality rate is 30% to 40%.

Type 4 infections are fungal. They most often affect immunocompromised patients and this likely contributes to their rapid clinical course and high mortality (>47% in immunocompromised).

SPREAD

The most obvious way for the pathogen to enter the body is through a compromise of the skin

Table 5
Microorganisms causing necrotizing soft tissue infections

Types of Neuro-fibromatosis	Cause	Organisms	Clinical Progress	Mortality
Type I (70%–80% cases)	Polymicrobial/ synergistic often bowel derived	Mixed anaerobes and aerobes. Gas gangrene or clostridial myonecrosis is a subtype	More indolent, better clinical progress, easier to recognize clinically	Variable; depends on underlying comorbidities
Type II (20%–30% cases)	Often monomicrobial, skin or throat-derived	Usually Group A β-hemolytic streptococcus (GAS) and/or *Staphylococcus aureus*	Aggressive, protean presentations easily missed	>32%, depends if associated with myositis or toxic shock; 30%–40%
Type III (more common in Asia)	Gram-negative, often marine-related organisms	*Vibrio* spp mainly (salt water), *Aeromonas hydrophila* (fresh water)	Seafood ingestion or water contamination	30%–40%
Type IV (fungal)	Usually trauma associated, immunocompetent patients	*Candida* spp immuno-compromised patients. Zygomycetes immunocompetent patients	Aggressive with rapid extension especially in immuno-compromised	>47% (higher if immunocompromised)

Adapted from Table 1 of Morgan MS. Diagnosis and management of necrotising fasciitis: a multiparametric approach. J Hosp Infect. 2010;75(4):249-57.

Table 6
Factors conferring a predisposition to specific extremity necrotizing soft tissue infections

Predisposing Factor	Clinical Syndrome	Etiologic Agent
Major penetrating trauma	Gas gangrene	*Clostridium* spp
Minor penetrating trauma • Freshwater • Saltwater	Type II	*Aeromonas hydrophila* *Vibrio vulnificus*
Minor nonpenetrating trauma	Type II	*Streptococcus pyogenes*
Skin breach • Varicella lesions • Insect bites • Injection drugs	Type II Type II Gas gangrene	*S pyogenes* *S pyogenes* *Clostridium* spp
Immunocompromised • Diabetes with peripheral vascular disease • Cirrhosis and ingestion of raw oysters • Neutropenia	Type I Type II Gas gangrene	Mixed aerobic and anaerobic *V vulnificus* *Clostridium septicum*

Adapted from Table 1 of Stevens DL, Bryant AE. Necrotizing Soft-Tissue Infections. N Engl J Med. 2017;377(23):2253-65.

such as trauma. However, this often does not exist, and it is then presumed that there was hematogenous seeding. Once the bacteria are present, they begin to spread along fascial planes. The bacteria release toxins causing vessels to clot. This combined with direct trauma of the invading organism results in tissue necrosis and encourages further spread of the pathogen.

The rate of progression of the disease depends on the type of pathogen as well as host factors. Toxins from the organisms have local effects that encourage their proliferation such as reducing blood flow and causing issue necrosis but also have systemic effects such as increasing endothelial permeability and decreasing vascular tone that can lead to cardiovascular collapse. They also impede the immune system by reducing phagocyte function. A unique characteristic of clostridial infections is myonecrosis not usually seen in other forms of NSTI. GAS have many additional characteristics that increase their pathogenicity, but a main factor is their ability to act as a superantigen and to create a massive cytokine cascade leading to toxic shock syndrome.

Treatment

Broad spectrum antibiotics should be started immediately if NSTI is suspected (**Fig. 4**). Based on the Infectious Disease Society of America, empirical treatment should be guided by the microbiologic classification of the suspected NSTI and further tailored with results of cultures and sensitivities.[38] GAS and clostridial NSTI should be treated with penicillin and clindamycin. Clindamycin is important, as it is effective at reducing alpha-toxin production clostridium species and the M protein production of the GAS. The synergistic effect with penicillin is that penicillin protects against GAS resistance to clindamycin. Vancomycin covers against *S aureus*. If suspected *V vulnificus* infection, then a combination of doxycycline and ceftriaxone or cefotaxime is effective. If type 4 infection is suspected, antifungal medications should be used.

There is some controversy about the duration of the antibiotics, but it is generally recommended that they should be continued until the infection is controlled and the patient is stable for 48 to 72 hours.[39]

Surgical Debridement

Prompt aggressive surgical debridement is the standard of treatment of NSTI, as it is the only form of treatment shown to reduce mortality. To emphasize, delayed and/or inadequate debridement greatly increases mortality rates for NSTI.[5,6,8,14,15] The goals are to reduce bacterial load and arrest tissue necrosis. In addition, tissue specimens and cultures can be obtained to further guide medical management.

Debridement must be aggressive and should include all affected tissues (skin, fascia, and muscle if involved) and should include a margin of healthy tissue, as the true extent of the infection is hard to delineate especially when dealing with a hyperacute case of NSTI.[6,19,22] A discrepancy between involvement of the skin, which may seem healthy, and the underlying involved fascia is a frequent finding. Surgical incisions must be designed for an extensile approach. Within the upper extremity, being aware of deep space infections such as involvement of the deep palmar space or even Parona space is crucial, and incisions should be made accordingly.

Multiple investigators have described tissue resistance being a useful guide to the extent of debridement. They note healthy tissue as requiring instruments to dissect, whereas finger pressure can easily create a tissue plane in necrotic tissues. As described earlier, consistent findings of NSTI are brownish, necrotic subcutaneous fat, "dishwater" fluid, lack of resistance to blunt dissection, as well as lack of bleeding tissue due to thrombosis of subcutaneous vessels.[10,16,21,22] It is crucial to control the infection proximally first to prevent further proximal spread and the associated increased risk for mortality.[21] Wounds should be left open and packed after the first debridement (Fig. 3). Drains or wound vacuum-assisted closure devices can be placed at the surgeon discretion, but the surgeon should plan on early return to the operating room within 24 hours.[16] The exact timing decision is made on the quality of the initial debridement and the clinical appearance of the patient. In addition, it should be planned to perform multiple debridements. Multiple studies[3,5–8,21] showed that on average 3 debridements were required.

A unique component of treatment of NSTIs in the hand and wrist is that amputation is a potential treatment and a surgeon should always be prepared for this possible intervention.[13] Although amputation of the upper extremity is less common than amputation of the lower extremity for NSTI, many studies use amputation as a treatment of upper extremity involvement.[3,5–8,19,21] Factors that contribute to the need for amputation include large area of tissue necrosis including underlying muscle, vascular insufficiency to the limb, or high anesthetic risk, as amputation is usually a quicker procedure with less blood loss.[21] It is notable that amputation does not increase survival,[6,21] and with many NSTIs, the infection does not spread deep to the fascia or compromise perfusion.[19] Consideration of amputation should include the survival of the patient and eventual morbidity of the amputation.

Once the patient is clinically stable and the wounds are cleared of infection and necrosis, then potential reconstructive procedures are considered. Often, more than one reconstructive procedure will be required.[3,8] Reconstructive procedures primarily involve skin grafting, but rotational flaps or other coverage procedures may be needed.[3] Skin grafts are limited by the amount of donor site tissues that are available as well as the location of wounds. The use of skin graft substitutes likely has benefit in reconstructive efforts especially with large areas of skin deficit.

Adjunctive Treatment

In addition to aggressive surgical debridement and antibiotic treatment, there are other modalities that can improve patient outcomes. Most importantly, the use of a multidisciplinary team is mandatory.[36,40] These patients often have systemic illness and require close monitoring. They require intensive supportive care in the form of

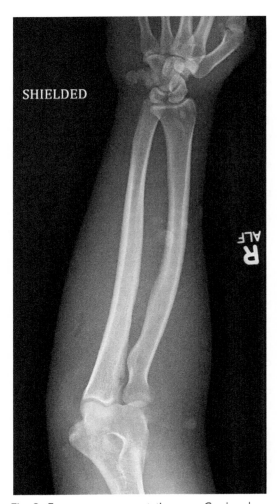

Fig. 3. From same representative case. Gas in subcutaneous tissues noted at the ulnar proximal forearm. Superficial blistering also noted.

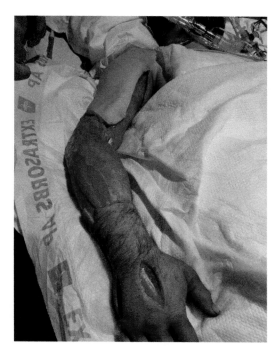

Fig. 4. Representative case. After initial series of debridement.

fluid resuscitation as well as metabolic and blood pressure support. Even after the infection has been controlled, the patient will require optimization of caloric intake, wound care, and reconstructive procedures. The multidisciplinary team includes critical care specialists, infectious disease specialists, plastic/reconstructive surgeons, wound care, nutritional support, nursing, other ancillary services, and the coordination of these services.

There are other treatments that can be used, one of which is the use of negative pressure wound therapy (NPWT). The use of NPWT is not well supported in the current literature on NSTI, but it is well supported in the literature regarding wound healing in various settings such as soft tissue defects and open fractures.[41] It is best to use NPWT once the infection is controlled and all necrotic tissues have been removed.[29] Some investigators believe that NPWT could exacerbate an infection,[41] so caution about the use of NPWT should be used if the infection is not clearly controlled. Because there is frequently a need for additional debridement within the next 24 hours, the use of NPWT after the initial surgery is often not necessary. Benefits of NPWT include promotion of healing, decreased bacterial load, and reduced wound size.[42] NPWT also reduces patient discomfort, improves wound care efficiency, and eases

wound care demands on nursing/wound care teams.[23]

Another adjunctive therapy that can be considered is hyperbaric oxygen (HBO) therapy. Treatment of NSTI is one of the primary indications for HBO,[43] but there is debate as to its effectiveness.[4,16] HBO works by enhancing oxygenation to tissues theoretically, leading to many positive effects for the treatment of NSTI. Increased oxygenation enhances the ability of leukocytes to kill bacteria and increases tissue perfusion, which prevents further necrosis and improves antibiotic dispersion and effectiveness, lipid peroxidation, and free radical scavenging.[43] However, HBO is not widely accessible and is expensive.

IV immunoglobulin therapy has been used as an adjunctive treatment of NSTI because of the potential to neutralize the endotoxins of the bacteria and mediate the cytokine cascade. However, at this point, no strong evidence exists for its benefit.[40] Consideration of the therapy should be limited to critically ill patients with staphylococcal and/or streptococcal NSTIs.[4]

Outcomes

Despite a growing understanding of the pathophysiology of NSTI, improved surgical technique, and adjunctive treatments, the mortality remains high. Studies frequently cite overall mortality rates of 15% to 33.7%.[3,6–8,21,44] One study did identify that patients with more distal involvement of an extremity had lower mortality (8.3%) compared with proximal involvement (58.3%).[21] Even with survival, limb loss (9%–22.5%) is common and need for reconstructive surgeries is often necessary.[3,5–8,19,21,44] In addition, hospitalization is often prolonged.[3,11] Because of the paucity of research, there is no good long-term understanding of the functional outcomes of the surviving patients.

SUMMARY

NSTIs of the upper extremities are a surgical emergency. The spectrum of disease processes, the diverse and often insidious appearing nature at presentation, and the systemic effects add to the complicated nature of their diagnosis and treatment. There remains high morbidity and mortality despite medical advances. Early and aggressive surgical treatment is paramount, and amputation of the limb has not been shown to improve outcomes, and indications are not clearly defined. Lastly, the care of these patients requires a team of medical professionals to achieve optimal outcomes.

CLINICS CARE POINTS

- Diagnosis can be difficult, and a high index of suspicion must be maintained.
- Disproportionate pain (extent and severity) is often an initial clue as to the presence of NSTI.
- Hemodynamic instability in the setting of an otherwise more benign appearing infection must be recognized as evidence of more severe disease present.
- Aggressive surgical debridement including healthy appearing tissues is crucial to arrest the pathogenesis of the disease.
- Surgery should never be delayed for additional tests or imaging if NSTI is highly suspected.
- Amputation does not improve patient outcomes but may be necessary.
- Expect to perform multiple debridements, with the second being within the next 24 hours.

DISCLOSURE

The authors have nothing to disclose

REFERENCES

1. Chauhan A, Wigton MD, Palmer BA. Necrotizing fasciitis. J Hand Surg Am 2014;39(8):1598–601 [quiz: 1602].
2. Anaya DA, McMahon K, Nathens AB, et al. Predictors of mortality and limb loss in necrotizing soft tissue infections. Arch Surg 2005;140(2):151–7 [discussion: 158].
3. Angoules AG, Kontakis G, Drakoulakis E, et al. Necrotising fasciitis of upper and lower limb: a systematic review. Injury 2007;38(Suppl 5):S19–26.
4. Hakkarainen TW, Kopari NM, Pham TN, et al. Necrotizing soft tissue infections: review and current concepts in treatment, systems of care, and outcomes. Curr Probl Surg 2014;51(8):344–62.
5. McHenry CR, Piotrowski JJ, Petrinic D, et al. Determinants of mortality for necrotizing soft-tissue infections. Ann Surg 1995;221(5):558–63 [discussion: 563-555].
6. Wong CH, Chang HC, Pasupathy S, et al. Necrotizing fasciitis: clinical presentation, microbiology, and determinants of mortality. J Bone Joint Surg Am 2003;85(8):1454–60.
7. Horn DL, Shen J, Roberts E, et al. Predictors of mortality, limb loss, and discharge disposition at admission among patients with necrotizing skin and soft tissue infections. J Trauma Acute Care Surg 2020;89(1):186–91.
8. Elliott DC, Kufera JA, Myers RA. Necrotizing soft tissue infections. Risk factors for mortality and strategies for management. Ann Surg 1996;224(5):672–83.
9. Cheng NC, Su YM, Kuo YS, et al. Factors affecting the mortality of necrotizing fasciitis involving the upper extremities. Surg Today 2008;38(12):1108–13.
10. Espandar R, Sibdari SY, Rafiee E, et al. Necrotizing fasciitis of the extremities: a prospective study. Strategies Trauma Limb Reconstr 2011;6(3):121–5.
11. Lemsanni M, Najeb Y, Zoukal S, et al. Necrotizing fasciitis of the upper extremity: a retrospective analysis of 19 cases. Hand Surg Rehabil 2021;40(4):505–12.
12. Schecter W, Meyer A, Schecter G, et al. Necrotizing fasciitis of the upper extremity. J Hand Surg Am 1982;7(1):15–20.
13. Uehara K, Yasunaga H, Morizaki Y, et al. Necrotising soft-tissue infections of the upper limb: risk factors for amputation and death. Bone Joint J 2014;96-B(11):1530–4.
14. Corona PS, Erimeiku F, Reverte-Vinaixa MM, et al. Necrotising fasciitis of the extremities: implementation of new management technologies. Injury 2016;47(Suppl 3):S66–71.
15. Bilton BD, Zibari GB, McMillan RW, et al. Aggressive surgical management of necrotizing fasciitis serves to decrease mortality: a retrospective study. Am Surg 1998;64(5):397–400. discussion: 400-391].
16. Stevens DL, Bryant AE. Necrotizing Soft-Tissue Infections. N Engl J Med 2017;377(23):2253–65.
17. Childers BJ, Potyondy LD, Nachreiner R, et al. Necrotizing fasciitis: a fourteen-year retrospective study of 163 consecutive patients. Am Surg 2002;68(2):109–16.
18. Gonzalez MH, Nikoleit J, Weinzweig N, et al. Upper extremity infections in patients with the human immunodeficiency virus. J Hand Surg Am 1998;23(2):348–52.
19. Gonzalez MH, Kay T, Weinzweig N, et al. Necrotizing fasciitis of the upper extremity. J Hand Surg Am 1996;21(4):689–92.
20. Roy S, Ninkovic J, Banerjee S, et al. Opioid Drug Abuse and Modulation of Immune Function: Consequences in the Susceptibility to Opportunistic Infections. J Neuroimmune Pharmacol 2011;6(4):442–65.
21. Tang WM, Ho PL, Fung KK, et al. Necrotising fasciitis of a limb. J Bone Joint Surg Br 2001;83(5):709–14.
22. Abrams RA, Botte MJ. Hand Infections: Treatment Recommendations for Specific Types. J Am Acad Orthop Surg 1996;4(4):219–30.
23. Choueka J, De Tolla JE. Necrotizing Infections of the Hand and Wrist: Diagnosis and Treatment Options. J Am Acad Orthop Surg 2020;28(2):e55–63.

24. Wall DB, Klein SR, Black S, et al. A simple model to help distinguish necrotizing fasciitis from nonnecrotizing soft tissue infection. J Am Coll Surg 2000; 191(3):227–31.

25. Wong CH, Khin LW, Heng KS, et al. The LRINEC (Laboratory Risk Indicator for Necrotizing Fasciitis) score: a tool for distinguishing necrotizing fasciitis from other soft tissue infections. Crit Care Med 2004;32(7):1535–41.

26. Wang TL, Hung CR. Role of tissue oxygen saturation monitoring in diagnosing necrotizing fasciitis of the lower limbs. Ann Emerg Med 2004;44(3): 222–8.

27. Chao WN, Tsai SJ, Tsai CF, et al. The Laboratory Risk Indicator for Necrotizing Fasciitis score for discernment of necrotizing fasciitis originated from Vibrio vulnificus infections. J Trauma Acute Care Surg 2012;73(6):1576–82.

28. Holland MJ. Application of the Laboratory Risk Indicator in Necrotising Fasciitis (LRINEC) score to patients in a tropical tertiary referral centre. Anaesth Intensive Care 2009;37(4):588–92.

29. Leiblein M, Marzi I, Sander AL, et al. Necrotizing fasciitis: treatment concepts and clinical results. Eur J Trauma Emerg Surg 2018;44(2):279–90.

30. Tsai YH, Hsu RW, Huang KC, et al. Laboratory indicators for early detection and surgical treatment of vibrio necrotizing fasciitis. Clin Orthop Relat Res 2010;468(8):2230–7.

31. Zacharias N, Velmahos GC, Salama A, et al. Diagnosis of necrotizing soft tissue infections by computed tomography. Arch Surg 2010;145(5): 452–5.

32. Martinez M, Peponis T, Hage A, et al. The Role of Computed Tomography in the Diagnosis of Necrotizing Soft Tissue Infections. World J Surg 2018; 42(1):82–7.

33. McGillicuddy EA, Lischuk AW, Schuster KM, et al. Development of a computed tomography-based scoring system for necrotizing soft-tissue infections. J Trauma 2011;70(4):894–9.

34. Kim KT, Kim YJ, Won Lee J, et al. Can necrotizing infectious fasciitis be differentiated from nonnecrotizing infectious fasciitis with MR imaging? Radiology 2011;259(3):816–24.

35. Koshy JC, Bell B. Hand Infections. J Hand Surg Am 2019;44(1):46–54.

36. Morgan MS. Diagnosis and management of necrotising fasciitis: a multiparametric approach. J Hosp Infect 2010;75(4):249–57.

37. Giuliano A, Lewis F Jr, Hadley K, et al. Bacteriology of necrotizing fasciitis. Am J Surg 1977;134(1):52–7.

38. Stevens DL, Bisno AL, Chambers HF, et al. Practice guidelines for the diagnosis and management of skin and soft tissue infections: 2014 update by the Infectious Diseases Society of America. Clin Infect Dis 2014;59(2):e10–52.

39. Bonne SL, Kadri SS. Evaluation and Management of Necrotizing Soft Tissue Infections. Infect Dis Clin North Am 2017;31(3):497–511.

40. Peetermans M, de Prost N, Eckmann C, et al. Necrotizing skin and soft-tissue infections in the intensive care unit. Clin Microbiol Infect 2020; 26(1):8–17.

41. Banwell PE, Musgrave M. Topical negative pressure therapy: mechanisms and indications. Int Wound J 2004;1(2):95–106.

42. Hu J, Goekjian S, Stone N, et al. Negative Pressure Wound Therapy for a Giant Wound Secondary to Malignancy-induced Necrotizing Fasciitis: Case Report and Review of the Literature. Wounds 2017;29(8):E55–60.

43. Greensmith JE. Hyperbaric oxygen therapy in extremity trauma. J Am Acad Orthop Surg 2004; 12(6):376–84.

44. Kumar T, Kaushik R, Singh S, et al. Determinants of Mortality in Necrotizing Soft Tissue Infections. Hell Cheirourgike 2020;92(5):159–64.

Shoulder and Elbow

Management of Acute Rotator Cuff Tears

Midhat Patel, MD[a], Michael H. Amini, MD[b],*

KEYWORDS

• Rotator cuff • Tear • Repair • Acute • Traumatic

KEY POINTS

- Rotator cuff tears in younger patients are more likely to be traumatic, most commonly due to a fall on an outstretched extremity or a glenohumeral dislocation.
- When there is suspicion of an acute, traumatic rotator cuff tear, advanced imaging is recommended to determine the extent and chronicity of injury.
- The current standard of care in young, active patients with full-thickness acute rotator cuff tears is operative repair, with earlier repair leading to better outcomes.
- There is controversy over the management of acute, full-thickness rotator cuff tears in low-demand patients.
- The current standard of care for acute, traumatic partial thickness rotator cuff tears is conservative management including physical therapy, activity modification, and intraarticular or subacromial injections.

INTRODUCTION

Shoulder pain is a common complaint, accounting for approximately 4.5 million office visits per year in the United States and affecting an estimated 8% of the adult population.[1,2] There are few studies in the literature that specifically address acute, traumatic rotator cuff tears, which are considered a different entity than the more commonly encountered degenerative tears (Fig. 1). One reason for this is that it is difficult to differentiate acute traumatic tears from an exacerbation of a previously existing degenerative tear secondary to an injury. The few studies that have sought to evaluate only acute traumatic tears use involvement of the subscapularis tendon and/or younger age as inclusion criteria, though this is controversial.[3]

There is no consensus in the literature on what defines an acute, traumatic rotator cuff tear. The authors consider the onset of shoulder pain in a patient without pre-existing pain after an injury with clinical and imaging findings of a rotator cuff tear to be acute within 6 to 12 months of the injury. The most commonly defined injury mechanisms in the literature include fall onto an outstretched hand, forced external rotation to an abducted extremity (such as grabbing an object while falling), and glenohumeral dislocation.[3] We acknowledge that even with these criteria there will be patients who likely had pre-existing degenerative pathology with tear extension, but it is difficult to distinguish these patients from those with true acute tears.

PATIENT EVALUATION

Clinical History and Physical Examination

A thorough history is critical for evaluating patients who present with acute shoulder pain concerning rotator cuff tear. Patient age, functional status, and expectations are important to determine to appropriately counsel patients on treatment options. It is critical to ask patients if they have antecedent pain in the shoulder to

---

[a] Department of Orthopedics, University of Arizona College of Medicine – Phoenix, 1320 North 10th Street, Suite A, Phoenix, AZ 85006, USA; [b] Shoulder and Elbow Surgery, The CORE Institute, 18444 North 25th Avenue #210, Phoenix, AZ 85023, USA
* Corresponding author.
E-mail address: amini.michael@gmail.com

Orthop Clin N Am 53 (2022) 69–76
https://doi.org/10.1016/j.ocl.2021.08.003
0030-5898/22/© 2021 Elsevier Inc. All rights reserved.

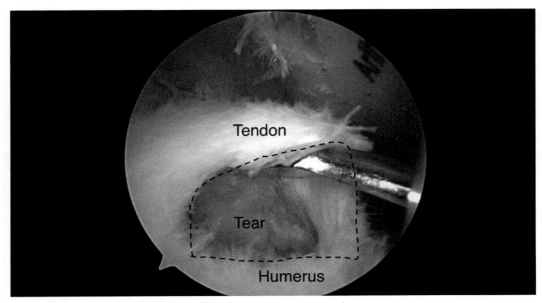

Fig. 1. Arthroscopic view of a rotator cuff tear. Dashed line outlining the tear.

distinguish between true acute tears versus further tearing of previous degenerative tears. In addition, the mechanism of injury should be discussed thoroughly to help determine potential pathologies.

A large variety of tests have been described for shoulder pathology, with different examinations used to determine what structures have been injured.[4] Described examination maneuvers are extensive and include the Neer sign, Hawkins sign, painful arc test, Jobe test, Full Can test, drop arm test, external rotation strength, Hornblower test, external rotation lag sign, belly press, belly-off, lift off, lift off lag sign, and bear hug, among others. Hippensteel and colleagues reviewed these examinations and reported specificity, sensitivity, and likelihood ratios.[5] They found that for the supraspinatus (SS), the painful arc test was the most useful as a screening tool, whereas the drop arm test was most useful as a confirmatory test. With respect to the infraspinatus (IS), external rotation weakness is sensitive while an external rotation lag sign is useful for confirmation. The Hornblower sign is effective in confirming injuries to the teres minor. Subscapularis pathology can be assessed with the belly-off test, which has high sensitivity and specificity.

The authors recommend using a combination of tests to evaluate for possible rotator cuff injury with evaluation of the contralateral upper extremity for comparison. Our assessment includes inspection for obvious muscle wasting, deformity, or evidence of previous surgery. This is followed by palpation to identify location of the patient's pain. We then carefully evaluate passive and active range of motion with attention to pain or limitation. This is followed by resisted elevation, external rotation, and internal rotation. Patients who have findings concerning acute rotator cuff tear such as pain and/or weakness with overhead motion, internal rotation, or external rotation are then referred for advanced imaging.

Imaging

Plain radiographs are obtained at the first visit after patients present with acute shoulder pain and a traumatic mechanism. They can be helpful in identifying pathology related to acute rotator cuff tears or other etiologies, and several signs can help suggest specific pathologies[6]:

- The presence of cortical irregularity or fracture of the greater tuberosity
- Enthesophytes or osteophytes in the subacromial space
- Calcification within the rotator cuff insertion or subacromial space
- Acromioclavicular joint arthritis
- Superior migration of the humeral head

In patients with suspected acute rotator cuff tears, MRI is the authors' preferred modality and should be obtained to evaluate the status of the rotator cuff tendons and musculature as well as possible concomitant injuries. MRI can be used to determine tear size, shape, depth, tendon involvement, and retraction to help guide treatment options (**Fig. 2**).[7] It is important to evaluate the periscapular musculature for evidence of fatty infiltration (**Fig. 3**), suggesting a more chronic injury that has been aggravated versus an acute tear.

Ultrasound is growing in popularity to evaluate the rotator cuff in patients with a suspected injury. It has been shown to have high specificity and sensitivity, equivalent to MRI in the diagnosis of rotator cuff tears.[8] The authors believe this is a useful screening modality in patients with a possible tear and an equivocal examination, especially if it can be done in the initial patient visit at the office; however, now, it is not able to replace MRI as it is limited in its ability to help diagnose concomitant pathologies around the shoulder or characterize muscular changes important to guiding appropriate treatment.

MR arthrography is also used for imaging of the shoulder with high sensitivity and specificity in diagnosing rotator cuff tears.[8] The authors do not recommend routine use of MR arthrography except in cases in which ultrasound and standard MRI are inconclusive. CT arthrography has also been used; however, it is not as

accurate as MRI or ultrasound for rotator cuff imaging. The authors do not recommend using CT arthrography unless the patient has a contraindication to MRI and ultrasound is equivocal with a suspected rotator cuff injury.[6]

TREATMENT
Nonoperative Management
Acute partial-thickness tears or small, full-thickness tears (<10 mm) in low-demand patients can be managed conservatively. Conservative management includes rest, activity modification, physical therapy, oral pain medications, or injections with corticosteroids or nonsteroidal anti-inflammatory drugs (NSAIDs).[9,10] Significant functional improvement has been shown with nonoperative treatment of partial-thickness tears.[11]

The current Clinical Practice Guidelines from the AAOS for management of rotator cuff tears have a moderate recommendation for initial treatment of cuff-related symptoms in the absence of a full tear with exercise/therapy and/or oral NSAIDs.[12] Baumer and colleagues[13] prospectively evaluated 25 patients with rotator cuff tears who underwent 8 weeks of physical therapy and compared them with matched controls that did not have tears. They found that therapy improved clinical outcomes, pain, range

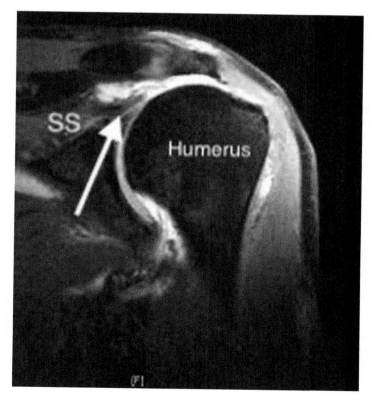

Fig. 2. MRI of a rotator cuff tear. Coronal T2-weighted MRI showing a tear of the supraspinatus. The arrow shows torn supraspinatus tendon edge.

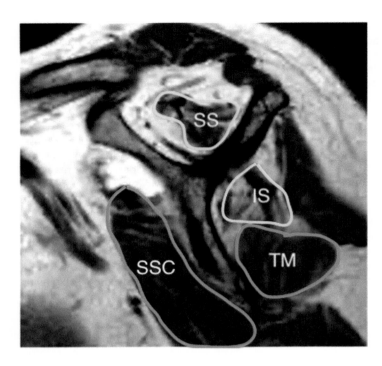

Fig. 3. MRI of a chronic rotator cuff tear. Sagittal T1-weighted MRI showing high-grade fatty infiltration in the SS and IS, with normal musculature in the SSC and TM. SSC, subscapularis; TM, teres minor.

of motion, and strength although not to the level of the control group. Kuhn reviewed 11 randomized-controlled trials which strongly suggested that physical therapy strongly improves pain and function associated with subacromial pain.[14] No difference was noted between formal physical therapy or home exercises.

There is a significant amount of literature dedicated to evaluating the effect of corticosteroid injections in rotator cuff disease. Multiple review articles have found that there is short-term benefit with pain relief compared to placebo or therapy alone.[15–17] However, it is important to note that they are not without risk—there are risks of cartilage damage, further tendon degeneration, detrimental effects to tendon healing, and risk of infection with future surgical procedures.[17] It is important to discuss with patients that surgical repair should be delayed after cortisone injection because of increased risk of infection and retear if done too close to the injection. There is conflicting evidence regarding the exact length of time repair should be delayed—large database studies examining incidence of infection after cortisone injection for arthroscopic shoulder procedures have shown 1 and 3 months as important time frames to delay surgery.[18,19] In addition, there is evidence to suggest that preoperative cortisone injections can increase the risk of failure of repair if done within 6 months of surgery.[20]

Subacromial anti-inflammatory injections have been shown to provide pain relief for patients with pain secondary to subacromial impingement.[10,21] Min and colleagues[10] performed a randomized controlled trial comparing intraarticular ketorolac (NSAID) versus triamcinolone and found improved clinical outcome scores, strength, and range of motion in the NSAID group at 4-week follow-up.

There is limited comparative data comparing acute, full-thickness, small rotator cuff tears treated operatively and nonoperatively. In a randomized controlled trial with 12 months follow-up, Ranebo and colleagues[22] showed that in patients with acute tears with a mean of 9.7 mm, there was no difference in clinical or functional outcome scores. However, they noted that 29.2% of unrepaired patients had tear progression of greater than 5 mm and 33% developed fatty infiltration. This is a major concern with nonoperative treatment of full-thickness tears: the risk of tear progression and muscle degeneration.

Although it is generally agreed upon that rotator cuff tears increase in size over time, there is minimal data regarding the risk of progression and natural history of acute, full-thickness small tears treated nonoperatively. Safran and colleagues[23] prospectively followed up patients younger than 60 years with a full-thickness tear >5 mm diagnosed on ultrasound. They found that of 61 tears, 49% had increased in size and that this correlated with an increase in pain. They concluded that patients in this population should be considered candidates for operative repair, and if treated nonoperatively, they should be monitored for tear progression. In contrast, Fucentese and colleagues[24] followed up 24 patients with full-thickness SS tears that were recommended to undergo surgical repair but declined. These patients had a mean age of 52 years. At an average follow-up of 3.5 years, they found no increase in the average tear size and slight progression of fatty atrophy with "surprisingly high" patient satisfaction. In both these studies, it is important to note that there is no mention of injury mechanism and how this could affect tear progression. However, they follow-up patients who are younger, and this may correlate to higher likelihood of acute versus degenerative tears.

We recommend initial conservative management for patients with acute, partial-thickness tears. Operative intervention can be considered for patients who fail conservative treatment.

We recommend that for patients with acute, full-thickness tears smaller than 10 mm, surgeons consider age and activity level when weighing the risks and benefits of operative repair and discussing this with patients. It is unclear whether or not surgery provides a definitive benefit in every case. For those who are treated nonoperatively, we recommend follow-up imaging at 12 to 18 months to monitor for tear progression.[11]

Operative

Acute, full-thickness tears larger than 10 mm (and smaller than 10 mm in young, active patients) should undergo operative repair within 4 months of injury (**Fig. 4**).[11,12] Based on limited data about the natural history of these tears, there is a high likelihood of tear progression without operative repair, including increase in tear size and fatty degeneration of the muscle bulk.[23] In addition, these tears tend to occur in younger patients and have a higher rate of healing than degenerative tears in older patients.[3,25,26]

Namdari and colleagues[27] reported outcomes in a series of 30 consecutive patients who underwent an open repair of traumatic anterosuperior rotator cuff tears with a mean follow-up of 56 months. They found that 29 of 30 patients were satisfied with their outcome, with shoulder function restored to nearly the same as the contralateral side. Moosmayer and colleagues[28] reported outcomes after 10-year

follow-up on patients with small to medium (<3 cm) full-thickness rotator cuff tears randomized to surgery or no surgery. They found that patients who underwent surgical repair had improved function, higher clinical outcome measures, and decreased pain compared with those treated nonoperatively. They also found that the magnitude of the difference between groups increased over time when compared with 1- and 5-year data.[29,30] It is important to note that this study did not separate between patients with acute and degenerative rotator cuff tears.

Several authors have examined the importance of timing and acuity of repair after traumatic rotator cuff tears, with conflicting results. Basset and Cofield[31] found that patients who underwent repair within 3 weeks of injury had better motion and less pain than those who had later surgery. Similarly, Hantes and colleagues[32] found comparable functional outcomes but better range of motion in patients who underwent repair within 3 weeks. Petersen and Murphy[33] examined outcomes in 36 patients who underwent repair and found no difference between 0 to 2 months and 2 to 4 months, but worse outcomes in patients who had surgery after 4 or more months. Björnsson and colleagues[26] found that for patients who underwent repair within 3 months, there was no difference in outcomes at any time point when broken down within the 3 months period.

In a larger study, Gutman and colleagues[34] retrospectively evaluated 206 patients with a minimum of 24 months follow-up who underwent repair of traumatic rotator cuff tears. They found that patients who underwent repair within 4 months had significantly better results than those who underwent later surgery. Subgroup analysis revealed improved pain and functional outcome scores in patients repaired within 3 weeks.

We recommend that for acute full-thickness rotator cuff tears larger than 10 mm (and smaller than 10 mm in young, active patients), surgical repair be performed with relative urgency as soon as possible (ideally within 3 weeks) and should not be delayed more than 4 months from the time of injury, if possible.

FUTURE DIRECTIONS

Significant resources are being applied to study the effects of various biologic augments such as platelet-rich plasma (PRP), human growth hormone (HGH), and collagen patches.[35] The current AAOS Clinical Practice Guidelines for

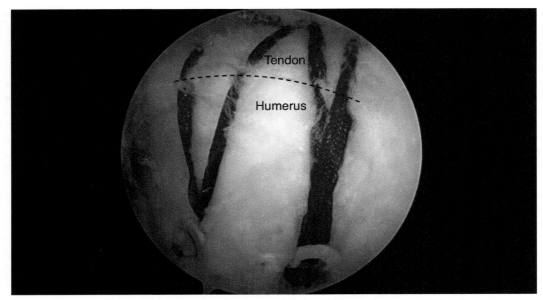

Fig. 4. Arthroscopic view of a rotator cuff repair. The dashed line shows the bone-tendon interface.

these interventions are in favor of liquid platelet-derived products, the use of dermal allografts in large-to-massive rotator cuff tears, and recommend against the use of xenografts.[9]

In a review of 18 level 1 studies, PRP was shown to decrease postoperative retear rates in tears involving multiple tendons, regardless of leukocyte number. There was also a statistically significant improvement in several clinical outcome measures across multiple studies; however, this did not reach a level of minimal clinically important difference for any of these measures.[36]

In a multicenter randomized controlled trial, Barber and colleagues[37] examined the use of acellular human dermal allograft matrix as an augment for tears greater than 3 cm at an average of 24 months follow-up. They found improved clinical outcome measures as well as increased rate of healing in patients in the augmented group. In another study looking at structure augmentation, Cai and colleagues[38] randomized patients with rotator cuff tears that had failed conservative treatment to repair with or without a 3D collagen matrix. They found no difference in clinical outcomes at final follow-up (mean 28.2 months) but a lower retear rate in the augmented group.

Oh and colleagues[39] randomized patients to receive weekly recombinant HGH (rHGH) injections for 3 months after repair of large (3–5 cm) posterosuperior cuff tears. They found no significant difference in patients with or without rHGH with respect to healing rates, range of motion, or pain.

At this time, there is not sufficient evidence to recommend the routine use of biologic or structural augments with surgical repair of traumatic rotator cuff tears. PRP and patch augments may be considered on an individual basis and discussed with patients.

SUMMARY

Patients presenting with symptoms concerning rotator cuff tear after a traumatic injury should undergo prompt assessment and imaging to evaluate the extent of the tear. Partial-thickness tears and small (<10 mm) full-thickness tears in low-demand patients can be managed conservatively with rest, activity modification, therapy, medications, and injections. Small full-thickness tears in high-demand patients and tears larger than 10 mm in most patients should be repaired operatively as soon as possible, within 4 months of injury at the latest. PRP and structural grafts may be considered to augment repair in individual cases.

CLINICS CARE POINTS

- Patients with a traumatic mechanism and pain or weakness with shoulder abduction and external rotation are at risk of having sustained an acute rotator cuff tear.

- Clinicians should have a low threshold for ordering MRI in patients suspected to have an acute rotator cuff tear.
- Partial-thickness rotator cuff tears and small tears (<10 mm) in low-demand patients can be treated conservatively with physical therapy, medications, and injections.
- Intraarticular anti-inflammatory medications are an effective alternative to cortisone, which may have detrimental effects and should be used with caution, especially in patients who may undergo future surgical repair.
- In full-thickness tears treated nonoperatively, imaging at 12 to 18 months is recommended to evaluate for tear progression. Attention should be paid to tear size, superior migration of the humeral head, and fatty infiltration.
- Full-thickness acute rotator cuff tears in active patients and full-thickness tears greater than 10 mm in all patients are at high risk of progression and should undergo operative repair.
- Outcomes of repair for traumatic cuff tears are best when performed within 3 weeks of injury, with significantly worse outcomes after 4 months.
- There is evidence to support PRP and structural grafts in specific patients and tear patterns and these can be discussed with patients and used on a case-by-case basis.

DISCLOSURE

M. Patel has nothing to disclose. M.H. Amini is a consultant to Stryker and FX Shoulder.

REFERENCES

1. Mather RC, Koenig L, Acevedo D, et al. The societal and economic value of rotator cuff repair. J Bone Joint Surg 2013;95(22):1993–2000.
2. Narvy SJ, Didinger TC, Lehoang D, et al. Direct cost analysis of outpatient arthroscopic rotator cuff repair in medicare and non-medicare populations. Orthop J Sports Med 2016;4(10). 2325967116668829.
3. Mall NA, Lee AS, Chahal J, et al. An evidenced-based examination of the epidemiology and outcomes of traumatic rotator cuff tears. Arthrosc J Arthrosc Relat Surg 2013;29(2):366–76.
4. Murrell GA, Walton JR. Diagnosis of rotator cuff tears. Lancet 2001;357(9258):769–70.
5. Hippensteel KJ, Brophy R, Smith MV, et al. A comprehensive review of physical examination tests of the cervical spine, scapula, and rotator cuff. J Am Acad Orthop Sur 2019;27(11):385–94.
6. Nazarian LN, Jacobson JA, Benson CB, et al. Imaging algorithms for evaluating suspected rotator cuff disease: society of radiologists in ultrasound consensus conference statement. Radiology 2013; 267(2):589–95.
7. Morag Y, Jacobson JA, Miller B, et al. MR imaging of rotator cuff injury: what the clinician needs to know1. Radiographics 2006;26(4):1045–65.
8. Jesus JO de, Parker L, Frangos AJ, et al. Accuracy of MRI, MR arthrography, and ultrasound in the diagnosis of rotator cuff tears: a meta-analysis. Am J Roentgenol 2009;192(6):1701–7.
9. Weber S, Chahal J. Management of rotator cuff injuries. J Am Acad Orthop Sur 2020;28(5):e193–201.
10. Min KS, Pierre PSt, Ryan PM, et al. A double-blind randomized controlled trial comparing the effects of subacromial injection with corticosteroid versus NSAID in patients with shoulder impingement syndrome. J Shoulder Elbow Surg 2013;22(5): 595–601.
11. Tashjian RZ. Epidemiology, natural history, and indications for treatment of rotator cuff tears. Clin Sport Med 2012;31(4):589–604.
12. Pedowitz RA, Yamaguchi K, Ahmad CS, et al. Optimizing the management of rotator cuff problems. Am Acad Orthop Surg 2011;19(6):368–79.
13. Baumer TG, Chan D, Mende V, et al. Effects of rotator cuff pathology and physical therapy on in vivo shoulder motion and clinical outcomes in patients with a symptomatic full-thickness rotator cuff tear. Orthop J Sports Med 2016;4(9). 2325967116666506.
14. Kuhn JE. Exercise in the treatment of rotator cuff impingement: a systematic review and a synthesized evidence-based rehabilitation protocol. J Shoulder Elb Surg 2009;18(1):138–60.
15. Gialanella B, Prometti P. Effects of corticosteroids injection in rotator cuff tears. Pain Med 2011; 12(10):1559–65.
16. Buchbinder R, Green S, Youd JM. Corticosteroid injections for shoulder pain. Cochrane Database Syst Rev 2003;2003(1):CD004016.
17. Coombes BK, Bisset L, Vicenzino B. Efficacy and safety of corticosteroid injections and other injections for management of tendinopathy: a systematic review of randomised controlled trials. Lancet 2010;376(9754):1751–67.
18. Werner BC, Cancienne JM, Burrus MT, et al. The timing of elective shoulder surgery after shoulder injection affects postoperative infection risk in Medicare patients. J Shoulder Elbow Surg 2016; 25(3):390–7.
19. Forsythe B, Agarwalla A, Puzzitiello RN, et al. The timing of injections prior to arthroscopic rotator cuff repair impacts the risk of surgical site infection. J Bone Joint Surg 2019;101(8):682–7.

20. Traven SA, Brinton D, Simpson KN, et al. Preoperative shoulder injections are associated with increased risk of revision rotator cuff repair. Arthrosc J Arthrosc Relat Surg 2019;35(3):706–13.

21. Itzkowitch D, Ginsberg F, Leon M, et al. Peri-articular injection of tenoxicam for painful shoulders: a double-blind, placebo controlled trial. Clin Rheumatol 1996;15(6):604–9.

22. Ranebo MC, Hallgren HCB, Holmgren T, et al. Surgery and physiotherapy were both successful in the treatment of small, acute, traumatic rotator cuff tears: a prospective randomized trial. J Shoulder Elbow Surg 2020;29(3):459–70.

23. Safran O, Schroeder J, Bloom R, et al. Natural history of nonoperatively treated symptomatic rotator cuff tears in patients 60 years old or younger. Am J Sports Med 2011;39(4):710–4.

24. Fucentese SF, Roll AL, Pfirrmann CWA, et al. Evolution of nonoperatively treated symptomatic isolated full-thickness supraspinatus tears. J Bone Jt Surg 2012;94(9):801–8.

25. Tashjian RZ, Hollins AM, Kim H-M, et al. Factors affecting healing rates after arthroscopic double-row rotator cuff repair. Am J Sports Med 2010; 38(12):2435–42.

26. Björnsson HC, Norlin R, Johansson K, et al. The influence of age, delay of repair, and tendon involvement in acute rotator cuff tears. Acta Orthop 2011; 82(2):187–92.

27. Namdari S, Henn RF, Green A. Traumatic anterosuperior rotator cuff tears. J Bone Jt Surg 2008;90(9): 1906–13.

28. Moosmayer S, Lund G, Seljom US, et al. At a 10-year follow-up, tendon repair is superior to physiotherapy in the treatment of small and medium-sized rotator cuff tears. J Bone Joint Surg 2019;101(12):1050–60.

29. Moosmayer S, Lund G, Seljom U, et al. Comparison between surgery and physiotherapy in the treatment of small and medium-sized tears of the rotator cuff. Bone Joint J 2010;92-B(1):83–91.

30. Moosmayer S, Lund G, Seljom US, et al. Tendon repair compared with physiotherapy in the treatment of rotator cuff tears. J Bone Jt Surg 2014; 96(18):1504–14.

31. Bassett RW, Cofield RH. Acute tears of the rotator cuff. Clin Orthop Relat R 1983;175(NA):18–24.

32. Hantes ME, Karidakis GK, Vlychou M, et al. A comparison of early versus delayed repair of traumatic rotator cuff tears. Knee Surg Sports Traumatol Arthrosc 2011;19(10):1766–70.

33. Petersen SA, Murphy TP. The timing of rotator cuff repair for the restoration of function. J Shoulder Elbow Surg 2011;20(1):62–8.

34. Gutman MJ, Joyce CD, Patel MS, et al. Early repair of traumatic rotator cuff tears improves functional outcomes. J Shoulder Elbow Surg 2021. https://doi.org/10.1016/j.jse.2021.03.134.

35. Tashjian RZ, Chalmers PN. What's new in shoulder and elbow surgery. J Bone Joint Surg 2019;101(20): 1799–805.

36. Chen X, Jones IA, Togashi R, et al. Use of platelet-rich plasma for the improvement of pain and function in rotator cuff tears: a systematic review and meta-analysis with bias assessment. Am J Sports Med 2019;48(8):2028–41.

37. Barber FA, Burns JP, Deutsch A, et al. A prospective, randomized evaluation of acellular human dermal matrix augmentation for arthroscopic rotator cuff repair. Arthrosc J Arthrosc Relat Surg 2012;28(1):8–15.

38. Cai Y-Z, Zhang C, Jin R-L, et al. Arthroscopic rotator cuff repair with graft augmentation of 3-dimensional biological collagen for moderate to large tears: a randomized controlled study. Am J Sports Med 2018;46(6):1424–31.

39. Oh JH, Chung SW, Oh K-S, et al. Effect of recombinant human growth hormone on rotator cuff healing after arthroscopic repair: preliminary result of a multicenter, prospective, randomized, open-label blinded end point clinical exploratory trial. J Shoulder Elbow Surg 2018;27(5):777–85.

Scapulothoracic Dissociation
A Review of an Orthopedic Emergency

Erick M. Heiman, DO[a], Jaclyn M. Jankowski, DO[b],
Richard S. Yoon, MD[b], John J. Feldman, MD[b],*

KEYWORDS

• Scapulothoracic dissociation • Orthopedic emergency • Treatment • Outcomes

KEY POINTS

• Scapulothoracic dissociation is a rare and often devastating injury.
• Thorough vascular and neurologic are mandatory in diagnosis.
• The amputation rate after these injuries ranges from 9% to 24%.
• Long-term sequelae are typically related to the degree of neurologic injury, with complete brachial plexus injuries having worse outcomes than incomplete injuries.
• Patients with a low likelihood of neurologic recovery benefit from early above-elbow amputation.

INTRODUCTION

Although rare, scapulothoracic dissociation (STD) is a devasting orthopedic injury that can potentially result in the loss of life or limb. Unfortunately, this extremely high-energy injury resulting from a distraction force on the upper extremity has a high propensity to be overlooked in the acute setting.[1] STD is a complex spectrum of injury that is currently defined as bony or ligamentous injury to the shoulder girdle, vascular injury to the subclavian or axillary vessels, brachial plexus injury, and severe soft-tissue disruption; analogous to an internal forequarter amputation.[2] Historically, this injury was described as complete disruption of the acromioclavicular joint with lateral displacement of the scapula, disruption of the subclavian vessels, and brachial plexus injury with the skin intact by Oreck and colleagues in 1987. This definition was subsequently modified by Ebraheim and colleagues in 1987[3,4] to include the entire shoulder girdle. This devastating injury carries with it a mortality rate of 11%. However, this is likely an underestimation given the high-energy mechanism and concomitant injuries that can cause death before reaching the hospital for diagnosis and evaluation.[4]

ANATOMY

It is important to understand the relevant osseous, muscular, and neurovascular anatomy that is potentially affected by STD. The scapula, which has no direct osseous attachment to the axial skeleton, interacts with the thorax via the infraserratus and supraserratus bursae. The scapula is further attached via the acromial clavicular (AC) joint to the clavicle, which is then attached to the axial skeleton via the sternoclavicular (SC) joint.[5] There are several muscle groups involved in the shoulder girdle's interaction with the axial skeleton, including the scapulothoracic, rotator cuff, and scapulohumeral muscles.[6]

The neurovascular anatomy of the upper extremity is important to understand when evaluating for STD. The arterial blood supply is

---

[a] Department of Orthopaedics, Jersey City Medical Center - RWJ Barnabas Health, 355 Grand St, Jersey City, NJ 07302, USA; [b] Jersey City Medical Center - RWJ Barnabas Health, 355 Grand St, Jersey City, NJ 07302, USA
* Corresponding author. 377 Jersey Avenue, Suite 280A, Jersey City, NJ 07302.
E-mail address: feldman.john@gmail.com

Orthop Clin N Am 53 (2022) 77–81
https://doi.org/10.1016/j.ocl.2021.08.004
0030-5898/22/© 2021 Elsevier Inc. All rights reserved.

redundant with collateral flow. The subclavian artery arises from the innominate artery on the right and the aortic arch on the left, with 5 main branches, becomes the axillary artery. The axillary artery has 6 main branches and terminates as the brachial artery over the anterior humeral shaft at the level of the inferior border of the teres major.[7,8] The nerve supply to the upper limb is supplied by the terminal branches of the brachial plexus, which originates from the C5-T1 nerve roots.[9]

PATHOGENESIS

STD occurs primarily through a high-energy mechanism of lateral traction to the upper limb, leading to a spectrum of severe osseous, vascular, and neurologic injuries. The osseous or ligamentous injury occurs within the shoulder girdle and can be an injury to the AC joint, SC joint, scapula, clavicle, or any combination thereof. A failure of the structural support leads to damage to local neurovascular structures. Associated vascular injury can lead to life-threatening internal hemorrhage or limb-threatening ischemic injury. Neurologic damage typically occurs as an avulsion injury to the brachial plexus. This can occur as either a preganglionic or postganglionic avulsion and often dictates the course of recovery. It is a combination of soft-tissue injuries that lead STD to act as an internal forequarter amputation.

DIAGNOSIS

STD should be suspected if the patient is known to have suffered a traction-type injury. On inspection, the entire shoulder girdle is typically swollen secondary to edema from the injuries or hematoma from the vascular injury. The injured upper extremity may be completely flaccid. A thorough vascular examination of the upper limb should be performed, beginning with palpation and doppler ultrasound evaluations of distal pulses.[10] Once the patient is determined to be hemodynamically stable and is able to participate in the examination, a thorough neurologic examination should be performed. Full sensory and motor examinations should be performed and compared to the contralateral side. It is important to determine preganglionic versus postganglionic injury to the brachial plexus. With a preganglionic injury, the patient will have weakness of the serratus anterior, rhomboids, and levator scapula; the patient may also present with Horner's syndrome (miosis, ptosis, anhidrosis).[11]

Initial imaging should consist of plain radiographs of the affected upper extremity as well as a well-centered chest radiograph (Fig. 1). A displaced clavicle fracture that is distracted more than 1 cm should place STD on the radar of the orthopedic team. Lateral displacement of the scapula is considered pathognomonic for STD and is quantified by the scapular index. The scapular index is assessed by measuring the distance between the medial border of the scapula and the thoracic spinous process, then obtaining the ratio between the injured and uninjured sides. A ratio of 1.29 or greater is diagnostic of STD.[12] If a diagnosis of STD is made on physical examination and initial radiographs, advanced imaging should be obtained. Computed tomography (CT) of the entire affected extremity should be obtained, along with angiography to assess vascular damage. In the setting of compete brachial plexus injury, Masmejean and colleagues advocate CT myelography within 3 weeks of the injury to confirm complete root avulsion and determine the level of injury. For incomplete brachial plexus injuries, they advocate MRI.[13]

CLASSIFICATION

The original classification of STD was described by Damschen and colleagues in 1997 and was based on the injured structures. Type 1 was isolated musculoskeletal injury. Type 2 was broken into 2 parts; type 2A was musculoskeletal injury with associated vascular injury, type 2B was musculoskeletal injury with associated incomplete neurologic impairment. Type 3 was a musculoskeletal injury with both vascular and incomplete neurologic injuries.[14] Zelle and colleagues revised the original classification in 2004 after evaluating the functional outcomes of the different types originally described by Damschen (Table 1). They found that patients with type 3 injuries did not have significantly worse outcomes than those with type 1 and type 2. They suggested an additional type 4 injury, which includes a musculoskeletal injury with complete brachial plexus avulsion, suggesting a complete neurologic injury and portends to significantly worse outcomes.[15]

TREATMENT

A universal treatment algorithm has not been settled on given the complex and rare nature of these injuries. Ebraheim and colleagues proposed a treatment protocol that is broken down into 3 phases encompassing the acute

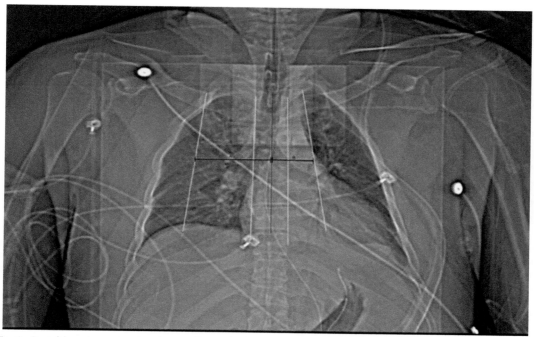

Fig. 1. Portable anteroposterior chest radiograph of a 42-year-old male obtained in the trauma bay after he suffered a motorcycle accident showing lateral displacement of the right scapula. Line A represents the distance from the spinous process to the medial border of the scapula of the injured side, line B represents the distance from the spinous process to the medial border of the scapula of the uninjured side. The scapular index is represented by A/B.

and chronic management of STD. Phase 1 involves the acute management of STD within the first 24 hours and is focused on limb salvage. Once stabilized, the patient is taken for exploration and repair of vascular injury, with concomitant osseous stabilization to protect the repair. The brachial plexus can be explored at this time and possibly grafted if appropriate. Phase 2 extends to the subacute period, within the next 2 weeks after the injury. During this phase, the decision is made whether to perform an above-elbow amputation in the setting of complete brachial plexus injury or irreparable skin/soft tissue injury, or to perform a shoulder arthrodesis. Phase 3 is considered the chronic phase and begins beyond 2 weeks after injury. During this phase, baseline nerve deficits are established with electromyography and necessary tendon or nerve transfers are performed. Continued monitoring can dictate further transfers as necessary, as well as prosthetic fit and occupational therapy for regain of function.[4]

Operative Intervention

The overall goal of operative intervention is creation of a vascularized limb with the best option for a painless functional upper extremity. When possible, the primary goal of function is to restore elbow flexion. Following initial revascularization and stability, there is a wide variety of operative interventions for STD, which are primarily dictated by the level and extent of brachial plexus injury.

Incomplete brachial plexus injuries, upper trunk injuries, typically demonstrate better outcomes than posterior cord injuries. Maldonado

Table 1 Damschen classification of scapulothoracic dissociation with Zelle modification	
Type	**Definition**
1	Musculoskeletal injury alone
2A	Musculoskeletal injury and vascular disruption
2B	Musculoskeletal injury and incomplete neurologic injury
3	Musculoskeletal injury with vascular disruption and incomplete neurologic injury
4	Musculoskeletal injury with complete brachial plexus avulsion

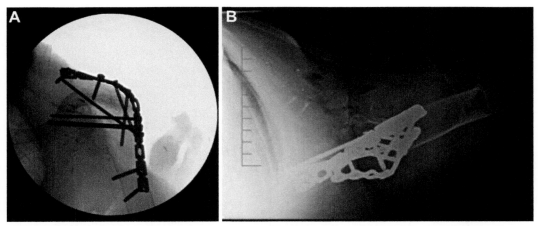

Fig. 2. (A) Intraoperative anteroposterior fluoroscopic view. (B) Postoperative axillary views of a patient 3 years after traumatic scapulothoracic dissociation with associated brachial plexus injury and multiple cervical nerve root avulsions. The patient developed a flail limb with arthrofibrosis. Multiple nerve transfers were attempted at an outside institution but were ultimately unsuccessful. Above-elbow amputation and shoulder arthrodesis were then indicated.

and colleagues reviewed procedures to restore function to upper trunk injuries and found that ulnar nerve fascicle transfer to biceps motor branch and triceps nerve fascicle transfer to axillary nerve provide excellent elbow flexion and shoulder abduction and external rotation. They found that posterior cord injuries led to inconsistent results with radial nerve grafting. Instead of nerve grafting these injuries, tendon transfers are recommended to restore function.[16]

Complete brachial plexus injuries are difficult to manage and often require more drastic operations to create a functional upper extremity. Dodakundi and colleagues described a 4-part process of double muscle transfer to restore elbow flexion and finger motion. This process was shown to have improved motor function and DASH scores compared to single free muscle transfer and nerve grafting alone.[17] Ultimately, this process requires brachial plexus exploration and repair within 5 months of injury, contralateral gracilis transfer to regain elbow flexion and finger extension, ipsilateral gracilis transfer to regain finger flexion, and all other indicated procedures to aid in these goals.[18] If a complete flail extremity is the likely outcome, the goal is to create a painless and functional upper extremity with primary above-elbow amputation, with or without primary shoulder arthrodesis (Fig. 2).

OUTCOMES

Long-term studies of STD demonstrate the devastating nature of this injury. A recent review by Branca and colleagues demonstrated that of those who survived the initial injury, 50% developed a flail limb and 20% eventually required an above-elbow amputation.[19] Damschen and Zelle reported a similar incidence of amputation of 21% to 24%.[14] With a more aggressive approach to early vascular repair, Reiss and colleagues demonstrated an amputation rate of 9%.[20] Although important for hemodynamic stability, it is unlikely that their aggressive vascular repairs lead to improved long-term outcomes, as overall outcomes are primarily dictated by the degree of brachial plexus injury.[21]

Long-term sequelae of STD are typically related to the degree of neurologic injury, and those with complete brachial plexus injuries have significantly lower Subjective Shoulder Rating System scores and SF-36 scores compared with those who have incomplete injuries.[15] Patients with complete brachial plexus injuries often are left with insensate, painful flail limbs, and without return of neurologic function at 6 months are unlikely to regain function.[22]

SUMMARY

Overall, STD is a rare and devastating injury that is considered an orthopedic emergency. It is critical to recognize this injury early based on mechanism, physical examination, and radiographic parameters. Initial management should be focused on resuscitation and evaluation for potential limb-threatening ischemia. Long-term outcomes are determined by the degree of neurologic injury, and patients with a low likelihood of neurologic recovery benefit from early above-elbow amputation.

CLINICS CARE POINTS

- Although rare, scapulothoracic dissociation is a devasting injury.
- Early diagnosis and treatment are essential.
- Treatment requires brachial plexus exploration and repair within 5 months of injury, contralateral gracilis transfer to regain elbow flexion and finger extension, ipsilateral gracilis transfer to regain finger flexion, and all other indicated procedures.
- Above-elbow amputation may be the best option for patients with little likelihood of neurologic recovery.

DISCLOSURE

The authors have nothing to disclose.

REFERENCES

1. Brucker PU, Gruen GS, Kaufmann RA. Scapulothoracic dissociation: evaluation and management. Injury 2005;36(10):1147–55.
2. Choo AM, Schottel PC, Burgess AR. Scapulothoracic dissociation: evaluation and management. J Am Acad Orthop Surg 2017;25(5):339–47.
3. Oreck SL, Burgess A, Levine AM. Traumatic lateral displacement of the scapula: a radiographic sign of neurovascular disruption. J Bone Joint Surg Am 1984;66(5):758–63.
4. Ebraheim NA, Pearlstein SR, Savolaine ER, et al. Scapulothoracic dissociation (closed avulsion of the scapula, subclavian artery, and brachial plexus): a newly recognized variant, a new classification, and a review of the literature and treatment options. J Orthop Trauma 1987;1(1):18–23.
5. Conduah AH, Baker CL, Baker CL. Clinical management of scapulothoracic bursitis and the snapping scapula. Sports Health 2010;2(2):147–55.
6. Wu JG, Bordoni B. Anatomy, Shoulder and Upper Limb, Scapulohumeral Muscle. [Updated 2021 Jan 18]. In: StatPearls [Internet]. Treasure Island (FL): StatPearls Publishing; 2021 Jan. Available at: https://www.ncbi.nlm.nih.gov/books/NBK546633/.
7. Bajzer C. Arterial supply to the upper extremities. In: Guide to peripheral and cerebrovascular intervention. London: Remedica; 2004. p. 124–34.
8. Thiel R, Munjal A, Daly DT. Anatomy, Shoulder and Upper Limb, Axillary Artery. [Updated 2021 Jul 26]. In: StatPearls [Internet]. Treasure Island (FL): StatPearls Publishing; 2021 Jan. Available at: https://www.ncbi.nlm.nih.gov/books/NBK482174/.
9. Ahimsadasan N, Reddy V, Kumar A. Neuroanatomy, Dorsal Root Ganglion. [Updated 2021 Jan 13]. In: StatPearls [Internet]. Treasure Island (FL): StatPearls Publishing; 2021 Jan. Available at: https://www.ncbi.nlm.nih.gov/books/NBK532291/.
10. Maria SW, Sapuan J, Abdullah S. The flail and pulseless upper limb: an extreme case of traumatic scapulo-thoracic dissociation. Malays Orthop J 2015;9(2):54–6.
11. Flanagin BA, Leslie MP. Scapulothoracic dissociation. Orthop Clin North Am 2013;44(1):1–7.
12. Doi K, Otsuka K, Okamoto Y, et al. Cervical nerve root avulsion in brachial plexus injuries: magnetic resonance imaging classification and comparison with myelography and computerized tomography myelography. J Neurosurg 2002;96(3 Suppl): 277–84.
13. Masmejean EH, Asfazadourian H, Alnot JY. Brachial plexus injuries in scapulothoracic dissociation. J Hand Surg Edinb Scotl 2000;25(4):336–40.
14. Damschen DD, Cogbill TH, Siegel MJ. Scapulothoracic dissociation caused by blunt trauma. J Trauma 1997;42(3):537–40.
15. Zelle BA, Pape H-C, Gerich TG, et al. Functional outcome following scapulothoracic dissociation. J Bone Joint Surg Am 2004;86(1):2–8.
16. Maldonado AA, Bishop AT, Spinner RJ, et al. Five operations that give the best results after brachial plexus injury. Plast Reconstr Surg 2017;140(3): 545–56.
17. Satbhai NG, Doi K, Hattori Y, et al. Functional outcome and quality of life after traumatic total brachial plexus injury treated by nerve transfer or single/double free muscle transfers: a comparative study. Bone Jt J 2016;98-B(2):209–17.
18. Dodakundi C, Doi K, Hattori Y, et al. Outcome of surgical reconstruction after traumatic total brachial plexus palsy. J Bone Joint Surg Am 2013;95(16): 1505–12.
19. Branca Vergano L, Monesi M. Scapulothoracic dissociation: a devastating "floating shoulder" injury. Acta Bio-Medica Atenei Parm 2018;90(1-S): 150–3.
20. Riess KP, Cogbill TH, Patel NY, et al. Brachial plexus injury: long-term functional outcome is determined by associated scapulothoracic dissociation. J Trauma 2007;63(5):1021–5.
21. Rorabeck CH, Harris WR. Factors affecting the prognosis of brachial plexus injuries. J Bone Joint Surg Br 1981;63-B(3):404–7.
22. Lavelle WF, Uhl R. Scapulothoracic dissociation. Orthopedics 2010;33(6):417–21.

Foot and Ankle

Compartment Syndrome of the Foot

Jeffrey S. Chen, MD, Nirmal C. Tejwani, MD*

KEYWORDS
• Compartment syndrome • Foot • Fasciotomy

KEY POINTS
• Foot compartment syndrome is an uncommon but debilitating condition typically resulting from high-energy fractures or crush injuries.
• Controversy exists regarding anatomic compartments, diagnosis, and treatment.
• The most objective method of diagnosis is direct measurement of compartment pressure.
• Both acute surgical intervention and delayed management can result in significant morbidity.

BACKGROUND

Foot compartment syndrome (FCS) is a debilitating but relatively uncommon condition accounting for approximately 3.5% of all limb compartment syndrome cases.[1] FCS is generally seen in the setting of high-energy injuries including crush and blast injuries, Chopart and Lisfranc fracture-dislocations, midfoot and forefoot trauma, and calcaneal fractures.[1–5] FCS has also been reported after tibial fracture both in isolation and concurrently with compartment syndrome of the leg, likely due to communication between the calcaneal compartment of the foot and the deep posterior compartment of the leg.[6,7]

The most common cause of FCS overall has traditionally been attributed to calcaneal fractures, with reports ranging from 3.8% to as high as 10% of cases.[8,9] These claims have recently been challenged by Thakur and colleagues who reviewed the National Trauma Data Bank and found that only 1% of patients (32 of 2481) with isolated calcaneal fractures underwent fasciotomy.[10] Thus, either the rate of FCS after calcaneal fractures is less than previously reported or FCS is underdiagnosed and undertreated. Their results showed that the highest incidence of FCS was seen with a crush injury combined with a forefoot injury (18%) or an isolated crush injury (14%) and an overall incidence of 2% after isolated trauma to the foot.[10]

The development of FCS is not limited to trauma. Any process that causes relative increases in compartment pressures can lead to FCS. This includes surgical procedures, occlusive dressings, vascular injuries and resulting ischemia/reperfusion syndromes, and overexertion.[7,11,12] Cases have also been reported of FCS after frostbite, snakebite, and inflammatory reactions.[13,14]

The recognition of FCS is important as severe long-term consequences can result if left untreated, including contractures, deformity, impaired ambulation, difficulty with footwear, and insensate feet with neuropathic pathology, all potentially resulting in chronic pain and disability.[2,3,7,15] Despite the serious repercussions of missed FCS, the relevant literature is sparse and controversies regarding both diagnosis and treatment persist.[16] The purpose of this review article is to compile the existing literature surrounding FCS and to summarize the current concepts regarding its management.

PATHOPHYSIOLOGY

Compartment syndrome results from increased pressure within a defined anatomic compartment bound by osseofascial planes with low

---

Department of Orthopedic Surgery, New York University Langone Orthopedic Hospital, NYU Langone Health, 301 East 17th Street, 14th Floor, New York, NY 10003, USA
* Corresponding author.
E-mail address: Nirmal.Tejwani@nyulangone.org

Orthop Clin N Am 53 (2022) 83–93
https://doi.org/10.1016/j.ocl.2021.08.005
0030-5898/22/© 2021 Elsevier Inc. All rights reserved.

compliance.[2,17] Increased pressure can result from either an increase in compartment contents, such as hemorrhage or edema, or from a decrease in compartment volume, such as use of tight casts, bandages, or splints. The typical presentation is a crush injury or fracture which results in continued hemorrhage and edema against the relatively inelastic surrounding connective tissue.[18] This increase in intracompartmental pressure leads to compromised perfusion and can culminate in permanent myoneural tissue damage if not released.

It is theorized that once compartment pressure exceeds capillary hydrostatic pressure, capillary collapse occurs and blood flow ceases.[15] Other proposed theories include arterial spasm following elevation of compartment pressure or collapse of arterioles once critical closing pressure within the compartment is reached.[19,20] Regardless of mechanism, the resultant stasis of blood flow induces a shift toward anaerobic metabolism. Oxygen debt can then induce increased capillary permeability and initiate inflammatory cascades, further increasing pressure and ultimately resulting in ischemia, soft tissue compromise, and necrosis.[21] Necrosis is then followed by fibrosis and contracture, leading to the late sequelae seen after untreated compartment syndrome.[15]

Muscle is particularly sensitive to changes in oxygen tension, with signs of dysfunction as early as 2 to 4 hours after ischemia and irreversible changes occurring at 4 to 12 hours.[22–24] Infarcted muscle undergoes a scarring process, which can progress for over 6 to 12 months after ischemic insult and result in significant contractures.[22] Neural deficits precede the onset of myoneural necrosis, but are still an intermediate finding as sensory changes do not occur until at least 30 minutes after the onset of ischemia.[2] Peripheral nerve damage may be irreversible after 4 to 6 hours.[25] Even after completion of the immediate process, continued muscle scarring can lead to late nerve compression and continued neural injury beyond the initial insult.[22] Chronic neuropathic symptoms can result, including numbness, neuropathic pain, allodynia, and hyperalgesia, and can result in chronic ulcers and joint destruction secondary to sensory disturbance.[3]

Both muscle and nerve injury can result in contracture formation. Common deformities following isolated FCS include toe deformity and pes cavus. Imbalance between the strong extrinsic muscles against the weak, scarred intrinsic foot muscles leads to deformities such as claw toe and hammertoe.[16] This can be exacerbated by an ischemic insult to the calcaneal compartment and the quadratus plantae, which inserts on the tendons of the flexor digitorum longus and can worsen flexion deformities with scarring.[22] Isolated neural injury leading to paralysis of the intrinsics is another possible cause. Cavus can result from scarring and contraction of plantar structures.[2] Compartment syndrome of the deep posterior compartment of the leg can also result in cavus. Combined FCS and compartment syndrome of the leg can create an even more complicated picture because of various combinations of imbalanced intrinsic and extrinsic muscle groups, leading to equinus, equinovarus, pes planus, and foot drop in addition to the aforementioned deformities.[22]

ANATOMY

The human foot is a complex anatomic structure. The exact number of compartments and their boundaries is controversial and has been debated extensively in the literature.[26] Early anatomic studies divided the foot into 4 compartments: medial, lateral, central, and interosseous.[27] Subsequent studies described varying combinations of 3 compartments: medial, lateral, and central versus intermediate.[28,29] In 1990, Manoli and Weber were prompted to investigate the compartments of the foot in greater detail after treating 3 patients with calcaneal fractures who later developed sequelae of FCS.[12] They conducted a cadaver study using dye injection and described a total of 9 compartments in the foot: medial, lateral, superficial, adductor, 4 interossei, and calcaneal.[12] This 9-compartment model has been widely adopted as the standard of clinical practice, despite several additional anatomic studies which have been published since their description.[30,31] Some have suggested the presence of a 10th dorsal compartment bounded by skin, containing the extensor digitorum brevis and extensor hallucis brevis.[32] The accuracy and clinical relevance of a potential compartment bounded by skin rather than fascia is unclear.

A recent systematic review collected 10 studies that evaluated the compartments of the foot and found a variety of methods, definitions, and conclusions, ranging from 3 to 10 compartments.[26] There was general agreement among authors regarding the presence of 3 major plantar compartments but less agreement regarding the dorsal foot. Only 2 studies were ranked with an overall low risk of bias, both of which agreed on 9 total compartments.[26]

Of the 9 compartments described by Manoli and Weber, 3 span the entire plantar aspect of the foot (medial, superficial, and lateral), 5 are confined to the forefoot (adductor and 4 interossei), and 1 is confined to the hindfoot (calcaneal) (Table 1). This was the first description of the calcaneal compartment, which has since been recognized as one of the most important compartments of the foot. The calcaneal compartment contains the quadratus plantae muscle, the lateral plantar neurovascular bundle, and in some patients, the medial plantar nerve.[17] It communicates proximally with the deep posterior leg compartment through the flexor retinaculum via the posterior tibial neurovascular bundle.[33] This has clinical relevance in the evaluation of the trauma patient with calcaneal fractures, tibial fractures, and/or crush injuries to either compartment as cases have been reported with combined compartment syndromes of the calcaneal and deep posterior leg compartments.[6] Because the calcaneal compartment is traversed by neurovascular bundles, severe disability can result if calcaneal compartment syndrome is untreated.[9] Studies have shown that the calcaneal compartment is subject to relatively higher pressures than other compartments.[12] This has been postulated to result from the large surface area of bleeding cancellous bone into the limited osseofascial compartment or from bleeding of the medial calcaneal artery into the quadratus plantae muscle.[9,34] Regardless of etiology, ischemia and contracture of the quadratus plantae and its insertion into the flexor digitorum longus tendon have been attributed to claw toe deformity.

CLINICAL PRESENTATION AND PHYSICAL EXAMINATION

The diagnosis of FCS is often less clear in comparison with compartment syndrome of the leg or upper extremity because of the complex anatomy and differences in relative muscle mass.[35] Pain, sensory, and motor changes are often not as impressive as findings in other locations.[18] For this reason, the examiner must maintain a high index of suspicion when evaluating for FCS with a low threshold for direct compartment pressure measurement if necessary. Classically taught findings of compartment syndrome include pain, poikilothermia, paresthesia, paralysis, pulselessness, and pallor.[36] In reality, the presence of most of these symptoms are late findings signaling irreversible damage to muscles and/or nerves. It is important to realize that compartment syndrome is an evolving process rather than a static one, and that changes in serial examinations are more meaningful than findings at a single time point.

Pain is the most common symptom of any patient presenting with a foot injury. Although all patients with FCS present with pain, those with crush injuries to the foot that do not develop FCS also present with severe pain. Therefore, the presence of pain itself cannot be used as a means of diagnosis. Pain in the presence of compartment syndrome is usually out of

Table 1
Nine compartments of the foot as described by Manoli and Weber

Location	Compartment	Contents
Full-Length Plantar[3]	Medial	Abductor hallucis Flexor hallucis brevis
	Lateral	Abductor digiti minimi Flexor digiti minimi brevis
	Superficial	Flexor digitorum brevis Flexor digitorum longus tendons Lumbricals (x4) +/− Medial plantar nerve, artery, vein
Forefoot[5]	Adductor	Adductor hallucis
	Interossei (x4)	Dorsal and plantar interossei
Hindfoot[1]	Calcaneal	Quadratus plantae Posterior tibial nerve, artery, vein Lateral plantar nerve, artery, vein +/− Medial plantar nerve, artery, vein

Data from Manoli A, 2nd, Weber TG. Fasciotomy of the foot: an anatomical study with special reference to release of the calcaneal compartment. *Foot Ankle.* 1990;10(5):267-275.

proportion to the injury and will not be relieved with adequate reduction and immobilization of the injured foot.[37] The presence of an open fracture does not rule out the possibility of a compartment syndrome as small fascial defects are unlikely to sufficiently relieve compartment pressures, let alone release all 9 compartments.[2,17] Progressively increasing analgesic requirement following extremity trauma should also heighten suspicion for developing FCS.[4]

Pain with passive stretch of an involved compartment is a common early finding before the onset of ischemia in compartment syndrome of the leg.[38] A similar finding can be seen with passive dorsiflexion of the toes in FCS. In a series of 14 cases of FCS, Myerson found that pain with passive dorsiflexion of the toes was present in 12 of 14 feet (85.7%).[37] In a similar series of 12 cases, Manoli and colleagues found only 6 of 12 feet (50.0%) to have pain with passive stretch.[6] The utility of this finding is questionable as passive toe dorsiflexion mostly involves the tendons of the long extrinsic flexor muscles of the leg.[16] In Manoli and colleagues' series, the most consistent finding was the presence of tense swelling, which was seen in all patients.[6]

Sensory changes are nonspecific findings that can be confounded by pain from the initial injury. Generally, decreased 2-point discrimination and light touch deficits on the plantar aspect and toes are more reliable than decreased pinprick sensation.[5] Relative changes with serial examinations are more sensitive than any single sensory examination. True neurologic findings are late findings and should be addressed with haste.

Assessment of vascular status is also not particularly helpful in the diagnosis of FCS. Palpable pulses are usually present at commonly tested sites (dorsalis pedis, posterior tibial) as they are extracompartmental.[7] Loss of palpable pulses would be a very late finding in compartment syndrome. Motor deficits are also not useful as strength is difficult to grade objectively and is often limited by pain.[5] Complete loss of motor innervation would again be a very late finding.

Given the ambiguous nature of the physical examination, most authors agree that compartment pressure measurement is the most reliable and objective method for diagnosing FCS.[2,3,18] A systematic review showed that in 95% of analyzed studies, surgical indication was based on either pressure measurements only or pressure measurements and clinical diagnosis.[39] Only 5% of all interventions were based on clinical examination alone.[39]

MEASURING COMPARTMENT PRESSURE

Examiners should have a lower threshold to resort to compartment pressure measurement than for the leg or upper extremity as the clinical picture of FCS is less certain. Some authors believe that compartment pressure measurement is the only means of reliably diagnosing FCS and recommend liberal use for any foot trauma with significant swelling.[5,40]

There are no set guidelines stating how many compartments or which compartments need to be measured when evaluating for FCS.[3,18] It is generally accepted that the calcaneal compartment must be measured if possible.[2] This is due to its relatively higher pressures, higher rates of involvement, and the compartment contents, which can lead to devastating sequelae if left untreated.[6,9]

Normal compartment pressures are usually less than 8 mm Hg.[21] Absolute compartment pressure greater than 30 mm Hg has been proposed as a cutoff for emergent decompression.[41] Animal studies have shown that pressures maintained above 30 mm Hg for 8 hours or longer can cause irreversible muscle and nerve damage.[42,43] Mittlmeier and colleagues studied 17 patients with calcaneal fractures and found that of the 12 patients with pressure measurements greater than 30 mm Hg, 7 patients (58.3%) had ischemic contractures after a mean follow-up of 18 months.[44] The 5 patients with pressures less than 30 mm Hg did not develop contractures.[44] A differential pressure (diastolic pressure − compartment pressure) less than 10 to 30 mm Hg is an alternative threshold for decompression.[45] This factors the presence of hypertension or hypotension into consideration, as is commonly seen in trauma patients.

Regardless of the method used, it is important to understand that no cutoff is perfectly sensitive and specific for the diagnosis of compartment syndrome. Patients have unique physiologic profiles and a compartment pressure leading to FCS in one patient may be tolerable in another. A more liberal cutoff will lead to more unnecessary fasciotomies, whereas a more conservative cutoff will lead to more missed compartment syndromes. In addition, recent studies have called into question the validity of pressure measurements as a whole, citing measurement inaccuracies, observer discrepancies, and lack of consensus as potential issues.[46] However, until more precise and consistent modalities are developed, pressure measurements are the most objective and widely available tests for the evaluation of compartment syndrome. The surgeon must incorporate the clinical picture with compartment measurements in their decision to proceed with intervention.

Compartments are measured using commercially available pressure monitors. The medial compartment is measured by inserting the needle approximately 4 cm inferior to the tip of the medial malleolus over the abductor hallucis muscle (**Fig. 1A**).[2] The needle can then be advanced into the calcaneal compartment. Reach and colleagues conducted a high-resolution MRI study of the compartments of the foot and recommended an entry point approximately 60 mm plantar to the most prominent aspect of the medial malleolus.[47] The needle is inserted approximately 10.75 mm deep to measure the medial compartment and then advanced to a total depth of approximately 24.33 mm deep to measure the calcaneal compartment.[47]

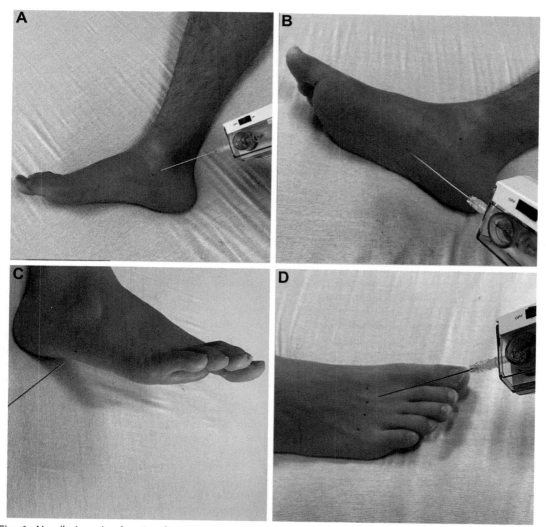

Fig. 1. Needle insertion location for measurement of foot compartments. (*A*) Medial compartment pressure is measured by inserting the needle approximately 4 cm inferior to the tip of the medial malleolus over the abductor hallucis muscle. The calcaneal compartment pressure is measured by advancing the needle 2 to 3 cm deep. (*B*) Superficial compartment pressure is measured by inserting the needle into the arch of the foot, penetrating the flexor digitorum brevis. (*C*) Lateral compartment pressure is measured by inserting the needle inferior to the fifth metatarsal. (*D*) The interosseous compartment pressures are measured by inserting the needle directly into the interosseous compartments dorsally. The adductor compartment is measured by advancing the needle deep to the interosseous compartments.

The superficial compartment is measured by inserting the needle into the arch of the foot, thereby penetrating the flexor digitorum brevis (Fig. 1B). The needle is then inserted just inferior to the fifth metatarsal to measure the lateral compartment (Fig. 1C). The interosseous compartments are then measured with 4 separate measurements by inserting the needle dorsally directly into the interosseous compartments. Finally, the adductor compartment is measured by advancing the needle deep to the interosseous compartments (Fig. 1D).

TREATMENT

Unlike compartment syndrome of the leg or upper extremity, treatment of FCS remains controversial. Both surgical release and delayed management are associated with potential morbidity that must be considered. Untreated FCS can lead to contractures, deformity, impaired ambulation, difficulty with footwear, and insensate feet with neuropathic pathology.[2,3,39,48,49] Surgical release subjects the patient to additional surgeries with potential soft coverage issues and an increased risk of infection in the setting of treatment of underlying fractures.[50] No high-quality prospective studies have compared early surgical decompression with observation and delayed management of FCS. Bedigrew and colleagues retrospectively compared patients who underwent foot fasciotomies with matched controls who underwent delayed management and found no significant differences in the development of neuropathic pain, sensory or motor deficits, chronic pain, stiffness, or infection.[51] In addition, patients who received fasciotomy were significantly more likely to develop claw toes (50% vs 17%, $P = .03$) and underwent an average of 5.5 surgeries per patient compared to 4 surgeries per patient in the control group.[51] Regardless of the treatment plan, if FCS is suspected, initial management should consist of immediate removal of all tight dressings, elevation of the extremity to the level of the heart, and prevention of systemic hypotension while the diagnosis is made.[5]

Acute Surgical Decompression
Fasciotomy is the definitive treatment for acute FCS. Consistent with the numerous compartmental models of the foot that have been described, multiple surgical techniques have been used for their surgical release, including various combinations of plantar, lateral, and dorsal incisions.[15,33] With the discovery of the

calcaneal compartment and the description of the 9-compartmental model by Manoli and Weber, there was a shift to a 3-incision technique, which is currently the most commonly described method for decompressive fasciotomy.[12,33] This method consists of a medial plantar incision and 2 dorsal incisions. The medial, lateral, superficial, and calcaneal compartments can be released through the medial incision. The 4 interossei and adductor compartments are released through the dorsal incisions.

Alternative approaches include using an isolated dorsal approach, which avoids medial soft tissue compromise but cannot access the calcaneal compartment, and a single medial plantar incision, through which all compartments can theoretically be accessed.[15] Both these approaches require deep, often blind dissection to adequately release all compartments and are challenging.

Using the 3-incision technique, the medial incision starts at a point 4 cm anterior to the posterior aspect of the heel and 3 cm superior to the plantar surface (just anterior to the abductor hallucis origin) and extends distally parallel to the plantar surface for 6 cm, releasing the medial compartment (Fig. 2).[12] The abductor hallucis is then reflected superiorly to expose the intermuscular septum and the calcaneal compartment behind it. Care must be taken to protect the lateral plantar nerve and vessels just deep into the fascia. This septum is entered and extended along the length of the skin incision to release the calcaneal compartment until bulging of the quadratus plantae is seen. Care must also be taken at the distal end of this incision as the medial plantar nerve can sometimes be present at the distal end of the calcaneal compartment. Because of its communication with the deep posterior compartment of the leg, some authors have suggested that adequate release of the calcaneal compartment may require release of the distal tarsal tunnel through extension of the medial incision posteriorly.[2]

The medial compartment is then reflected superiorly to identify the superficial compartment laterally. This is opened longitudinally releasing the flexor digitorum brevis. Finally, the flexor digitorum brevis is retracted inferiorly to allow exposure of the medial aspect of the lateral compartment. This is released along its visible extent longitudinally until the abductor digiti quinti and flexor digiti minimi are visible (Fig. 3).

Dorsally, 2 longitudinal incisions are made located medial to the second metatarsal and lateral to the fourth metatarsal with care to leave

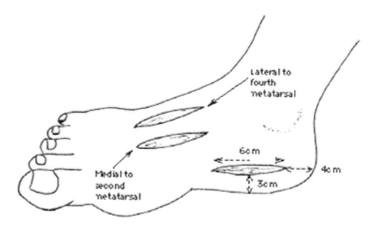

Fig. 2. Three-incision fasciotomy technique including 1 medial incision and 2 dorsal incisions. The medial incision allows access to the medial, superficial, calcaneal, and lateral compartments. The dorsal incision allows access to the interossei and adductor compartments. (*From* Fulkerson E, Razi A, Tejwani N. Review: acute compartment syndrome of the foot. *Foot Ankle Int.* 2003;24(2):180-187.; with permission.)

a sufficient skin bridge to avoid necrosis (see Fig. 2). This effectively releases the 4 interossei compartments. Finally, the interspace muscles from the medial aspect of the second metatarsal are elevated to expose the adductor compartment deep to the muscles. This is opened longitudinally, completing the fasciotomy (Fig. 4).

Fasciotomy incisions, especially medially based incisions, frequently require delayed closure or skin grafting. Wound closure is generally indicated 5 to 7 days postfasciotomy.[9] In the setting of fracture, it has been recommended that calcaneal fixation should be delayed due to risk of infection with exposed hardware,

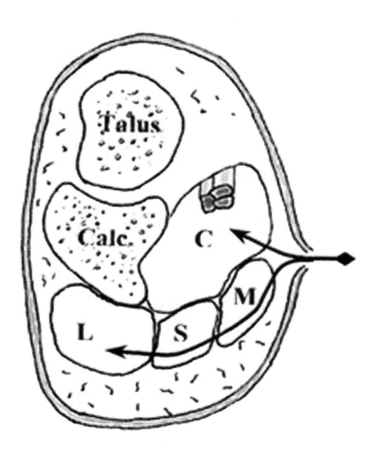

Fig. 3. Axial cross-sectional diagram demonstrating accessible compartments through the medial plantar incision of the 3-incision fasciotomy technique. Care must be taken to avoid the lateral and medial plantar neurovascular bundles while releasing these compartments. C, calcaneal; L, lateral; M, medial; S, superficial. (*From* Fulkerson E, Razi A, Tejwani N. Review: acute compartment syndrome of the foot. *Foot Ankle Int.* 2003;24(2):180-187.; with permission.)

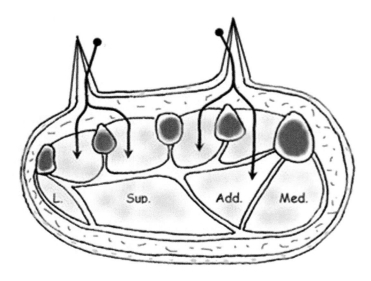

Fig. 4. Axial cross-sectional diagram demonstrating accessible compartments through the 2 dorsal incisions of the 3-incision fasciotomy technique. The adductor compartment is best accessed by dissecting deep into the first interosseous compartment. Add., adductor; L, lateral; Med., medial; Sup., superficial. (*From* Fulkerson E, Razi A, Tejwani N. Review: acute compartment syndrome of the foot. *Foot Ankle Int.* 2003;24(2):180-187.; with permission.)

whereas midfoot and forefoot fractures can be stabilized at the time of fasciotomy as long as the skin can be closed primarily.[9,40]

Wound closure issues and postoperative complications related to fasciotomy are not benign. Ojike and colleagues systematically reviewed the available data for 39 cases of FCS treated with fasciotomy and found that 20 of 31 patients (64.5%) required split-thickness skin grafts, 17 of 39 patients (43.6%) had contractures or neurologic complications, 15 of 39 patients (38.5%) had residual pain and stiffness, and only 4 of 26 patients (15.4%) were able to return to work.[39] Despite these results, the authors believe that the complications of fasciotomy are far outweighed by the complications of delayed treatment.[39] This review is limited by the variety of fasciotomy techniques that were used (ranging from 1 to 4 incisions) and lack of comparison to a delayed treatment group.

More recently, Han and colleagues reported slightly better results in their prospective study of 14 patients with FCS who underwent fasciotomy for an average follow-up of 24 months.[50] All patients underwent delayed wound closure, none developed wound infections, and 78.6% (11 of 14) returned to work. A shorter time to fasciotomy was correlated with improved functional scores, lower pain scores, and the ability to return to work. A total of 5 patients (35.7%) demonstrated FCS-related sequelae, 2 with claw toe deformity and 3 with persistent sensory deficits.[50]

Given the potential morbidities associated with fasciotomy, some authors have advocated

less invasive techniques such as dorsally based dermal fascial fenestrations, or "pie-crusting," in which multiple small incisions are made in an attempt to reduce soft tissue complications and promote wound healing (**Fig. 5**).[52,53] Lufrano and colleagues conducted a cadaver study comparing fasciotomy with dorsal dermal fascial fenestrations and found that fasciotomy was more effective in decreasing intracompartmental pressure.[54] Specifically, fenestrations were unable to effectively decompress the abductor (medial) and superficial plantar compartments and only partially decompressed the dorsal compartment.[54] However, the release of hematoma and swelling may decrease the pressure adequately in early diagnosis.

Ling and Kumar conducted a cadaver study and concluded that, contrary to previous studies, only 3 compartments of the foot exist and only 2 of them (intermediate and lateral) are completely encased in fascia requiring release.[30] They cite errors of previously conducted dye infusion and MRI studies and note that fascia was not found in many areas where previously reported. Based on their findings, they refute the 3-incision technique and instead recommend a single plantar incision on the non–weight-bearing instep of the foot starting 5 cm from the posterior edge of the heel and extending 5 cm distally. They state this approach is safer and provides all the relevant releases necessary for FCS.[30] Additional data are necessary to support the use of this approach in a clinical setting.

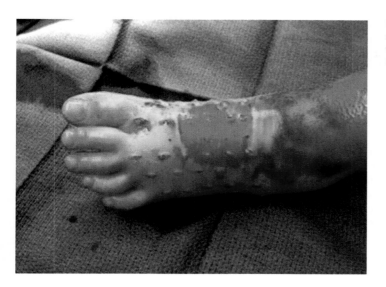

Fig. 5. Clinical photograph demonstrating dorsally based dermal fascial fenestrations, the "pie-crusting" technique.

Delayed Management and Reconstruction

Fasciotomy should not be performed if diagnosis of FCS has been delayed for more than 8 hours as the risk of local infection secondary to necrotic muscle outweighs the potential benefit.[18] Finkelstein and colleagues described 5 patients with a delayed diagnosis of FCS of more than 35 hours and found that 1 patient succumbed to multisystem organ failure while the remaining 4 required lower limb amputations secondary to infection.[55] Thus, for patients presenting late in the acute phase of FCS or in the chronic setting, fasciotomy should be avoided. Some surgeons choose to observe FCS even in the acute setting as they feel that the sequelae and their management are less morbid than fasciotomy.[1,3]

The goal of delayed management is to achieve a functional, plantigrade, and painless foot.[16] Initial management should aim to prevent contracture and preserve mobility. Passive mobilization, stretching therapy, and splinting are options for preventing contracture. Patients should have access to accommodative footwear options such as deep toe boxes for claw toe and orthotics for cavus foot, and should be educated about proper skin care and monitoring for ulceration if they have any insensate areas.[18] Chronic neuropathic pain is a potential sequelae, which is associated with decreased quality of life and psychosocial functioning.[56] Management is difficult and often requires a multidisciplinary approach with multimodal drug therapy.[57]

Surgical intervention may be indicated for those who have failed nonsurgical treatment.

Lesser toe deformities can be managed with a variety of surgical procedures. Soft tissue procedures can be used for flexible deformities, including flexor tendon tenotomy, extensor tendon lengthening, and flexor-to-extensor tendon transfer (Girdlestone-Taylor procedure).[48,49] For rigid deformity, arthrodesis with or without shortening osteotomies and metatarsophalangeal joint capsulectomies are recommended.[21] Cavus is managed first with soft tissue procedures such as scar excision, plantar fascia release, tendon transfers, and Achilles lengthening.[22] If inadequate, osteotomy and arthrodesis can be considered. In cases of concomitant cavus and claw toe deformity, transfer of the extensor digitorum longus to the metatarsal necks addresses both deformities.[3] Amputation is a salvage option for debilitating cases that are poor candidates for reconstruction and should not be considered a failure of treatment.[3]

SUMMARY

FCS is a relatively uncommon condition usually seen in the setting of high-energy crush injuries. Despite its debilitating consequences, controversy persists throughout all aspects of its management. The development of FCS is an evolving process that requires high clinical suspicion and serial examination. Direct compartment pressure measurement is currently the most objective method in the workup of FCS and should be incorporated with the clinical picture when making a diagnosis. The most accepted anatomic model of the foot at this time comprises 9 compartments, of which the calcaneal compartment carries the greatest risk of long-term deficits if left untreated. Management of FCS remains controversial as both surgical and nonsurgical treatments are associated with morbidity. Fasciotomy is the most effective surgical treatment and usually consists of a 3-incision technique; an alternative is the "pie-crusting" technique, which is less invasive. Nonoperative treatment will likely result in the sequelae of contractures, deformity, and neuropathy, which may require reconstruction at a later time. Further research is necessary regarding the outcomes of acute versus delayed intervention.

CLINICS CARE POINTS

- Clinical suspicion and early diagnosis of compartment syndrome are important when assessing high energy injuries to the foot.
- Compartment pressure monitoring is helpful in diagnosis.
- Adequate release and delayed closure of fasciotomy wounds are recommended.
- It may be helpful to use external fixation for fracture stabilization if needed.

DISCLOSURE

The authors have nothing to disclose.

REFERENCES

1. Middleton S, Clasper J. Compartment syndrome of the foot–implications for military surgeons. J R Army Med Corps 2010;156(4):241–4.
2. Fulkerson E, Razi A, Tejwani N. Review: acute compartment syndrome of the foot. Foot Ankle Int 2003;24(2):180–7.
3. Dodd A, Le I. Foot compartment syndrome: diagnosis and management. J Am Acad Orthop Surg 2013;21(11):657–64.
4. Shereff MJ. Compartment syndromes of the foot. Instr Course Lect 1990;39:127–32.
5. Myerson M. Diagnosis and treatment of compartment syndrome of the foot. Orthopedics 1990; 13(7):711–7.
6. Manoli A 2nd, Fakhouri AJ, Weber TG. Concurrent compartment syndromes of the foot and leg. Foot Ankle 1993;14(6):339.
7. Manoli A 2nd. Compartment syndromes of the foot: current concepts. Foot Ankle 1990;10(6):340–4.
8. Park YH, Lee JW, Hong JY, et al. Predictors of compartment syndrome of the foot after fracture of the calcaneus. Bone Joint J 2018;100-B(3):303–8.
9. Myerson M, Manoli A. Compartment syndromes of the foot after calcaneal fractures. Clin Orthop Relat Res 1993;(290):142–50.
10. Thakur NA, McDonnell M, Got CJ, et al. Injury patterns causing isolated foot compartment syndrome. J Bone Joint Surg Am 2012;94(11):1030–5.
11. Jowett A, Birks C, Blackney M. Chronic exertional compartment syndrome in the medial compartment of the foot. Foot Ankle Int 2008;29(8):838–41.
12. Manoli A 2nd, Weber TG. Fasciotomy of the foot: an anatomical study with special reference to release of the calcaneal compartment. Foot Ankle 1990;10(5):267–75.
13. Brandao RA, St John JM, Langan TM, et al. Acute compartment syndrome of the foot due to frostbite: literature review and case report. J Foot Ankle Surg 2018;57(2):382–7.
14. Hon KL, Chow CM, Cheung KL, et al. Snakebite in a child: could we avoid the anaphylaxis or the fasciotomies? Ann Acad Med Singap 2005;34(7):454–6.
15. Lutter C, Schoffl V, Hotfiel T, et al. Compartment Syndrome of the foot: an evidence-based review. J Foot Ankle Surg 2019;58(4):632–40.
16. Lugo-Pico JG, Aiyer A, Kaplan J, et al. Foot Compartment Syndrome Controversy. In: Mauffrey C, Hak DJ, Martin IM, editors. Compartment syndrome: a guide to diagnosis and management. 2019. p. 97–104. Cham (CH).
17. Matsen FA 3rd. Compartmental syndrome. An unified concept. Clin Orthop Relat Res 1975;(113):8–14.
18. Perry MD, Manoli A 2nd. Foot compartment syndrome. Orthop Clin North Am 2001;32(1):103–11.
19. Benjamin A. The relief of traumatic arterial spasm in threatened Volkmann's ischaemic contracture. J Bone Joint Surg Br 1957;39-B(4):711–3.
20. Burton AC. On the physical equilibrium of small blood vessels. Am J Physiol 1951;164(2):319–29.
21. Botte MJ, Santi MD, Prestianni CA, et al. Ischemic contracture of the foot and ankle: principles of management and prevention. Orthopedics 1996; 19(3):235–44.
22. Santi MD, Botte MJ. Volkmann's ischemic contracture of the foot and ankle: evaluation and treatment of established deformity. Foot Ankle Int 1995;16(6):368–77.
23. Hargens AR, Schmidt DA, Evans KL, et al. Quantitation of skeletal-muscle necrosis in a model compartment syndrome. J Bone Joint Surg Am 1981;63(4):631–6.
24. Vaillancourt C, Shrier I, Vandal A, et al. Acute compartment syndrome: how long before muscle necrosis occurs? CJEM 2004;6(3):147–54.

25. Ugalde V, Rosen BS. Ischemic peripheral neuropathy. Phys Med Rehabil Clin N Am 2001;12(2):365–80.

26. Vazquez-Zorrilla D, Millan-Alanis JM, Alvarez-Villalobos NA, et al. Anatomy of foot Compartments: a systematic review. Ann Anat 2020;229:151465.

27. Grodinsky M. A study of the fascial spaces of the foot and their bearing on infections. Surg Gyn Obstet 1929;49:737–51.

28. Kamel R, Sakla FB. Anatomical compartments of the sole of the human foot. Anat Rec 1961;140:57–60.

29. Feingold ML, Resnick D, Niwayama G, et al. The plantar compartments of the foot: a roentgen approach I. Experimental observations. Invest Radiol 1977;12(3):281–8.

30. Ling ZX, Kumar VP. The myofascial compartments of the foot: a cadaver study. J Bone Joint Surg Br 2008;90(8):1114–8.

31. Faymonville C, Andermahr J, Seidel U, et al. Compartments of the foot: topographic anatomy. Surg Radiol Anat 2012;34(10):929–33.

32. Reach JS Jr, Amrami KK, Felmlee JP, et al. Anatomic compartments of the foot: a 3-Tesla magnetic resonance imaging study. Clin Anat 2007;20(2):201–8.

33. Myerson MS. Experimental decompression of the fascial compartments of the foot–the basis for fasciotomy in acute compartment syndromes. Foot Ankle 1988;8(6):308–14.

34. Andermahr J, Helling HJ, Rehm KE, et al. The vascularization of the os calcaneum and the clinical consequences. Clin Orthop Relat Res 1999;(363):212–8.

35. Dayton P, Goldman FD, Barton E. Compartment pressure in the foot. Analysis of normal values and measurement technique. J Am Podiatr Med Assoc 1990;80(10):521–5.

36. Raza H, Mahapatra A. Acute compartment syndrome in orthopedics: causes, diagnosis, and management. Adv Orthop 2015;2015:543412.

37. Myerson MS. Management of compartment syndromes of the foot. Clin Orthop Relat Res 1991;(271):239–48.

38. Ulmer T. The clinical diagnosis of compartment syndrome of the lower leg: are clinical findings predictive of the disorder? J Orthop Trauma 2002;16(8):572–7.

39. Ojike NI, Roberts CS, Giannoudis PV. Foot compartment syndrome: a systematic review of the literature. Acta Orthop Belg 2009;75(5):573–80.

40. Fakhouri AJ, Manoli A 2nd. Acute foot compartment syndromes. J Orthop Trauma 1992;6(2):223–8.

41. Willy C, Sterk J, Volker HU, et al. [Acute compartment syndrome. Results of a clinico-experimental study of pressure and time limits for emergency fasciotomy]. Unfallchirurg 2001;104(5):381–91.

42. Hargens AR, Akeson WH, Mubarak SJ, et al. Fluid balance within the canine anterolateral compartment and its relationship to compartment syndromes. J Bone Joint Surg Am 1978;60(4):499–505.

43. Hargens AR, Romine JS, Sipe JC, et al. Peripheral nerve-conduction block by high muscle-compartment pressure. J Bone Joint Surg Am 1979;61(2):192–200.

44. Mittlmeier T, Machler G, Lob G, et al. Compartment syndrome of the foot after intraarticular calcaneal fracture. Clin Orthop Relat Res 1991;(269):241–8.

45. Whitesides TE, Haney TC, Morimoto K, et al. Tissue pressure measurements as a determinant for the need of fasciotomy. Clin Orthop Relat Res 1975;113:43–51.

46. Hak DJ, Mauffrey C. Limitations of pressure measurement. In: Mauffrey C, Hak DJ, Martin IM, editors. Compartment syndrome: a guide to diagnosis and management. 2019. p. 51–8. Cham (CH).

47. Reach JS Jr, Amrami KK, Felmlee JP, et al. The compartments of the foot: a 3-tesla magnetic resonance imaging study with clinical correlates for needle pressure testing. Foot Ankle Int 2007;28(5):584–94.

48. Perry MD, Manoli A 2nd. Reconstruction of the foot after leg or foot compartment syndrome. Foot Ankle Clin 2006;11(1):191–201, x.

49. Brey JM, Castro MD. Salvage of compartment syndrome of the leg and foot. Foot Ankle Clin 2008;13(4):767–72.

50. Han F, Daruwalla ZJ, Shen L, et al. A prospective study of surgical outcomes and quality of life in severe foot trauma and associated compartment syndrome after fasciotomy. J Foot Ankle Surg 2015;54(3):417–23.

51. Bedigrew KM, Stinner DJ, Kragh JF Jr, et al. Effectiveness of foot fasciotomies in foot and ankle trauma. J R Army Med Corps 2017;163(5):324–8.

52. Dunbar RP, Taitsman LA, Sangeorzan BJ, et al. Technique tip: use of "pie crusting" of the dorsal skin in severe foot injury. Foot Ankle Int 2007;28(7):851–3.

53. Poon H, Le Cocq H, Mountain AJ, et al. Dermal fenestration with negative pressure wound therapy: a technique for managing soft tissue injuries associated with high-energy complex foot fractures. J Foot Ankle Surg 2016;55(1):161–5.

54. Lufrano R, Nies M, Ebben B, et al. Comparison of dorsal dermal fascial fenestrations with fasciotomy in an acute compartment syndrome model in the foot. Foot Ankle Int 2019;40(7):853–8.

55. Finkelstein JA, Hunter GA, Hu RW. Lower limb compartment syndrome: course after delayed fasciotomy. J Trauma 1996;40(3):342–4.

56. Baron R, Binder A, Wasner G. Neuropathic pain: diagnosis, pathophysiological mechanisms, and treatment. Lancet Neurol 2010;9(8):807–19.

57. Macone A, Otis JAD. Neuropathic Pain. Semin Neurol 2018;38(6):644–53.

Temporizing Care of Acute Traumatic Foot and Ankle Injuries

Ivan S. Tarkin, MD[a],[*], Christopher D. Murawski, MD[b],
Peter N. Mittwede, MD, PhD[b]

KEYWORDS

- Lower extremity fractures • Foot and ankle injuries • External fixation • Staged management
- Temporizing fixation

KEY POINTS

- Severe foot and ankle injuries often have associated soft tissue damage that precludes immediate definitive surgical fixation.
- In severe injuries of the foot and ankle that are amenable to reconstruction, a staged surgical treatment approach is often necessary.
- The host, injury pattern, associated injuries, and surgeon resources should all be considered when deciding on the temporizing treatment of severe lower extremity trauma.
- Temporizing treatment of severe foot and ankle injuries should be individualized to the patient and injury pattern, but include splinting, external fixation, percutaneous reduction and/or fixation, and limited open reduction and internal fixation methods.

INTRODUCTION

Temporizing care has become a critical part of the treatment armamentarium for select foot and ankle injuries. Indications for performing temporizing care are based on the specific injury pattern, the host, associated injuries, as well as surgeon resources.[1] Foot and ankle injuries are often associated with severe adjacent injury to the soft tissue sleeve. An acute procedure performed through a traumatized soft tissue envelope will often lead to the failure of wound healing and/or infectious complications.[2,3] Thus, delayed reconstruction of acute foot and ankle injuries is often advisable in these cases.

The host must be considered when individualizing care for severe foot and ankle injuries. Temporizing care with delayed reconstruction is typically chosen for the patient with medical comorbidities, as these patients benefit from medical optimization before their open definitive surgical procedure.[4] Prehabilitation in these cases includes aggressive medical management of both acute and chronic illnesses.[5] Attention should also be given to improving nutrition as well as curbing any negative social behaviors such as drug, alcohol, or tobacco abuse.[6,7]

Severe foot and ankle injuries are often associated with other injuries to the musculoskeletal system, head, spine, chest, and/or abdomen. Acute definitive care of severe foot and ankle injuries in the setting of polytrauma is typically not practical or recommended. However, short- and long-term functional outcomes for the patient with multisystem injuries are often predicated on the successful treatment of their foot and ankle trauma.[8–10] Therefore, temporizing care is of paramount importance in this patient cohort until both host physiology and local soft tissue conditions allow for definitive reconstruction.

---

[a] Department of Orthopaedic Surgery, University of Pittsburgh, 3471 Fifth Avenue Suite 1010, Pittsburgh, PA 15213, USA; [b] Department of Orthopaedic Surgery, University of Pittsburgh, Pittsburgh, PA, USA
* Corresponding author.
E-mail address: tarkinis@upmc.edu

Orthop Clin N Am 53 (2022) 95–103
https://doi.org/10.1016/j.ocl.2021.09.002
0030-5898/22/© 2021 Elsevier Inc. All rights reserved.

Access to an orthopedic traumatologist or foot and ankle specialist is not always achievable when a patient presents with severe foot and ankle trauma requiring an operation. Further, hospital resources including personnel and equipment may not be readily available on the arrival of these patients. In these scenarios, temporization plays a critical role in slowing the cycle of injury to the foot/ankle before the planning and execution of the definitive care plan.[11] It is important for orthopedic surgeons taking call at smaller hospitals to be aware of their capabilities and resources, and when indicated, be prepared to perform temporizing procedures before transfer to a larger trauma center.

PATIENT EVALUATION AND DECISION MAKING

Understanding a patient's medical history, mechanism of injury, physical examination, imaging studies, and laboratory values are of paramount importance in deciding whether a definitive operation or temporizing care is appropriate for a particular foot and ankle injury. Specifically, a staged approach is typically favored in patients with medical problems that are associated with poor wound healing potential. For example, a conservative strategy with mindful delayed reconstruction is often chosen in patients with uncontrolled diabetes or significant peripheral vascular disease.[12]

There is a paucity of soft tissue coverage in the foot and ankle, in particular muscle, which predisposes this region to complications after injury and surgical intervention.[13] The physical examination is critical to determine whether there is threatened skin from bone and/or joint deformity. Further, the foot needs to be examined for both vascular and/or neurologic compromise that would require prompt attention. Temporizing care assumes a critical role in the correction and stabilization of the deformity to slow the ongoing injury to the soft tissue envelope as well as to the bone and joint surfaces.

Evaluation of swelling is a major determinant in deciding whether to proceed acutely with a definitive operation or staged care. The presence of fracture blisters is a sign of severe concomitant soft tissue injury. Serous or hemorrhagic blisters can be present, with hemorrhagic blisters indicating a more severe injury to the dermal-epidermal junction.[14] Surgeons should avoid placing a surgical incision through these areas, and should often wait until these have re-epithelialized before proceeding with definitive surgical management of foot and ankle fractures. In the absence of blistering, the "wrinkle sign" is an indicator of the degree of swelling and suitability for open surgical care.[15] When in doubt, temporizing care is warranted to avoid local complications.

Open foot and ankle injuries should most often be treated in a staged manner. By definition, these injuries are associated with severe insult to the soft tissues. In addition to debridement and irrigation, the skeletal and or joint injuries should be reduced and stabilized. The injury mechanism is a primary determinant of whether temporizing or definitive care should be performed. Specifically, it should be determined whether the mechanism of trauma was high or low energy. In high-energy cases, the soft tissue envelope is typically severely traumatized and posttraumatic swelling is expected. The maximal swelling typically occurs between days 2 and 7 after injury.[14] If the host and/or local soft tissues cannot tolerate the definitive open operation acutely, then staged management is chosen with plans for delayed reconstruction. Temporizing care must address fracture deformity and/or joint dislocation appreciated on injury films as well as effectively immobilize the bone and/or articular injury.

Imaging studies including orthogonal radiographs, computed tomography (CT), and less commonly magnetic resonance imaging (MRI) allow for the precise classification of the specific foot and ankle injury. The definitive surgical plan can be designed based on these data. To obtain a complete understanding of the local injury complex, imaging including the ipsilateral knee and tibia/fibula should be obtained, as well as other parts of the body whereby injuries are suspected. The decision to proceed with obtaining advanced imaging before versus after a potential temporizing operation depends on the type and severity of the bony and soft tissue injury. There are times when it is advisable to wait until after the temporizing procedure to obtain a CT scan to allow for improved understanding of the injury pattern when the bones are in a more anatomic position.[16,17] However, if there is any chance that definitive fixation will be performed acutely and the injury pattern merits advanced imaging, a CT scan should be obtained in the emergency department.

The use of laboratory values and vital signs as part of the patient evaluation is important when evaluating patients with polytrauma or comorbid medical conditions with foot and ankle injuries. Objective serum markers for nutrition and chronic illness, including (but not limited to) prealbumin, albumin, creatinine, hemoglobin, and hemoglobinA1C (HgA1C) are helpful in decision making. Markers of resuscitation are important when evaluating the polytrauma patient with foot and ankle trauma, including lactic acid, base deficit, and bicarbonate.[18] In chronically ill or under-resuscitated multisystem trauma patients, a staged approach with temporizing initial care is most appropriate.

SURGICAL TREATMENT OPTIONS
Temporizing care
Temporizing care of foot and ankle injuries can be delivered in a multitude of ways and should be tailored to the specific host, injury pattern, and circumstance (**Fig. 1**). Strategies for consideration include percutaneous pinning, external fixation, percutaneous reduction, and limited open reduction methods.

Percutaneous pinning can be used to temporize fractures or alternatively, transarticular pins can be used to stabilize unstable joints. Pin stabilization is used after closed or percutaneous manipulation or alternatively with a limited open reduction. A common application of this technique includes ankle/fracture dislocations in the form of a tibiotalocalcaneal Steinmann pin.[19] Chopart dislocations are frequently unstable and require pinning as a temporizing measure. Occasionally, talus fracture/dislocations

not amenable to acute open reduction internal fixation (ORIF) are pinned temporarily whereas awaiting soft tissue recovery. Midfoot dislocations and metatarsal fractures tenting the skin may also require temporary pin fixation.

External fixation is the "workhorse" for temporizing acute foot and ankle trauma as part of a staged management protocol. Placement of a frame causes minimal soft tissue disruption. This form of "traveling traction" allows for reduction via ligamentotaxis. As opposed to standard splinting, the frame allows for soft tissue monitoring as well as evaluation for compartment syndrome. External fixation for foot and ankle injuries can be tailored to the specific foot and ankle injury. Frames are composed of strategically placed Shantz pins combined with bars and clamps. Thin-tensioned wires can be used as well, either as part of a hybrid construct or a formal circular frame. The standard Ilizarov method or the more modern adjustable Taylor spatial method can be used, with these methods being effective for either staged or definitive management.[20,21]

If closed reduction is ineffective and even a limited open reduction is unsafe secondary to traumatized soft tissues, a percutaneous reduction of the fracture or dislocated foot and/or ankle should be considered. Schanz pins or taps can be inserted percutaneously to

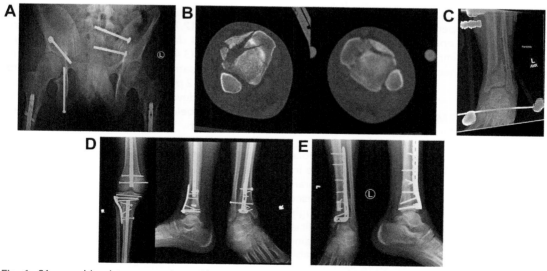

Fig. 1. 21-year-old polytrauma patient with numerous orthopedic injuries including combined pelvic/acetabular trauma (A), bilateral femur fractures, a left patella fracture, a right tibial plateau fracture, right segmental diaphyseal tibia fractures, a left olecranon fracture, and bilateral tibial pilon fractures (B; right AO/OTA 43B, left AO/OTA 43C) after a high-speed motor vehicle accident. On admission, the patient also presented with both chest and abdominal trauma. Damage control orthopedics was initiated using closed reduction and temporizing external fixation (C). Definitive fixation of the musculoskeletal injuries was deferred until the host physiology improved. Further, management of the bilateral tibial pilon fractures was performed after adjacent soft tissue injury had resolved (D, E).

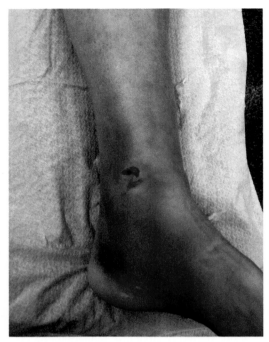

Fig. 2. Skin tenting and ultimate tissue necrosis after redislocation of a trimalleolar ankle fracture initially managed in a splint. Consideration for initial external fixation is warranted when delayed ORIF is necessary to avoid this complication.

"joystick" the fracture or dislocation into appropriate alignment (Fig. 2). Alternatively, percutaneously applied clamps can be considered. When limited open incisions are necessary, either to perform open fracture care or to obtain a reduction, it is important to consider the incisions that will be necessary for the definitive surgical procedure.

OUTCOMES - TEMPORIZING CARE FOR TIBIAL PILON FRACTURES

External fixation for pilon fractures has revolutionized the standard of care by which these injuries are managed. It allows for temporary fixation and staged reconstruction as opposed to acute definitive fixation, which is fraught with complications ranging from superficial wound issues to deep infection rates exceeding 35% in historical series.[2,3] Given unacceptably high complication rates with acute definitive fixation, external fixation techniques as well as hybrid external and limited internal fixation techniques have been studied. The articular blocks in higher-energy pilon injuries are frequently irreducible by ligamentotaxis alone and these techniques were, therefore, expectedly limited by

early posttraumatic arthritis in the setting of articular malunion.[22,23] The results from these series have encouraged the modern standard of care for staged treatment protocols.

Helfet and colleagues reported 34 high-energy pilon fractures in 32 patients, of which a small subset of 6 patients was treated in a staged fashion with temporizing external fixation as a means of optimizing soft tissue status before definitive fixation.[24] Two subsequent studies evaluated formal staged treatment protocols for tibial pilon fractures. Patterson and Cole retrospectively evaluated 21 consecutive patients with 22 type 43C pilon fractures treated with immediate fibular nailing and medial ankle-spanning external fixation.[25] At a mean of 24 days after the initial temporizing procedure, patients underwent delayed reconstruction and were followed for a mean 22 months. Seventy-seven percent of patients reported good outcomes using subjective and objective measurements, and no wound complications or infections were reported. In a separate study, Sirkin and colleagues identified 108 type 43C pilon fractures treated over a 6-year period, 56 of which were retrospectively evaluated as part of an analysis of staged treatment and the effect on surgical wound complications.[26] There were 34 closed fractures and 22 open fractures, all of which underwent ORIF of the fibula (when fractured) and application of an ankle-spanning external fixator within 24 hours of presentation. Definitive fixation was then possible after an average of 12.7 days in the closed fracture group and 14 days in the open fracture group. One patient (3.4%) developed osteomyelitis in the closed treatment group requiring hardware removal, and 2 patients (10.5%) in the open fracture group developed a deep infection, one requiring a below-knee amputation. A more recent study by Wang and colleagues randomly allocated 56 partial or complete articular pilon fractures to receive staged ORIF versus limited internal and external fixation and found that whereas clinical outcomes were similar, patients in the limited internal and external fixation group experienced higher superficial soft tissue infection rates.[27] From these studies, the use of temporizing fixation and delayed reconstruction can be advocated as the standard of care for minimizing soft tissue complications associated with high-energy pilon fractures.

More recent work has focused on optimizing care patterns when using staged treatment protocols. Ankle-spanning external fixation confers an opportunity to reestablish coronal and sagittal plane alignment, length, and rotation.[28,29] Care should be taken during external fixation to achieve these goals to avoid a more challenging second stage operation or revision procedure. In this regard, Barei and colleagues revealed in their review that 40 of 42 (95%) patients transferred to a tertiary trauma center required revision external fixation for a pilon fracture before definitive treatment, frequently secondary to tibial malreduction.[30] The optimal type of external fixator to use in complete articular pilon fractures has also been evaluated. Ramlee and colleagues performed a finite element analysis to determine the biomechanical stability of 3 different external fixators, including unilateral and Delta external fixators, as well as a Mitkovic frame.[31] Their model indicated that the Delta frame yielded the lowest relative micromovement (0.03 mm) during a stance phase of simulated gait, whereas the Mitkovic frame (0.05 mm) and unilateral fixator (0.42 mm) were appreciably higher. Therefore, Delta-type frames seem to be the most stable external fixator for type III pilon fractures. With respect to further optimizing construct stability, the addition of a first metatarsal pin can be considered. Recently, Albagli and colleagues retrospectively examined the addition of a first metatarsal pin to an ankle-spanning Delta frame in 37 patients by comparison to 30 patients who underwent Delta frame only.[32] The authors found that 20% of patients with the Delta frame and 18.9% who had an additional first metatarsal pin demonstrated some form of early loss of reduction ($P = .576$). Further investigation is required on the ideal frame type for pilon fractures.

The ideal placement of the calcaneal pin when applying an external fixator has been studied. Theoretically, the posteromedial tibial neurovascular bundle may be at risk, but Santi and Botte performed a study using 15 cadaver feet, and found that there was a large medial calcaneal safe zone on the posterior tuberosity located posterior to the neurovascular bundle and tendons.[33] The medial calcaneal nerve, the most posterior lateral plantar nerve, and the lateral and medial plantar nerves are also at risk with calcaneal pins, and a study by Casey and colleagues helped to highlight the safest areas for pin placement.[34]

Infection rates relating to definitive fixation methods and whether they overlap with external fixation pin sites have been studied. Shah and colleagues previously performed a retrospective comparative study including bicondylar tibial plateau fractures and type 43C pilon fractures who underwent staged management with external fixation, of whom 50 patients had overlapping pin sites and 132 did not.[35] The authors reported a 24% deep infection rate in the overlapping group and 10% rate in the group whereby pin sites did not overlap, which was statistically significant ($P = .033$). Despite this, however, several more recent studies by Potter and colleagues,[36] Hadeed and colleagues,[37] and Dombrowsky and colleagues[38] have disputed these findings. Dombrowsky and colleagues retrospectively evaluated 146 patients with high-energy pilon fractures over a 7-year period who underwent ankle-spanning external fixation and delayed ORIF.[38] Overlap of definitive plate and external fixation pins was noted in 40% of cases, of which 12% developed deep infection compared with 17% of patients without overlap ($P = .484$). These studies suggest that emphasis can be placed on placing temporizing external fixation pins to achieve the necessary construct stability as opposed to ensuring placement outside of the zone of definitive fixation.

Hardeski and colleagues examined the sterilization of external fixators for surgery in cases whereby it is desired that they be left in place for repeat operations.[39] Forty-eight patients with 55 external fixators were prospectively enrolled and prepped with sterile gloves and 70% alcohol-soaked gauze followed by standard skin preparation, after which cultures were obtained from 3 sites on each external fixator. Only 2 cultures were positive for pathogens commonly observed in surgical site infection, suggesting that a standard preparation protocol may be sufficient in producing an environment as clean as possible for external fixators already in place. Nielsen and colleagues found acceptable deep and superficial infection rates after definitive fixation when the external fixator was prepped into the surgical field.[40]

OUTCOMES - TEMPORIZING CARE FOR UNSTABLE ANKLE FRACTURES

The lessons learned from managing pilon fractures in a staged fashion have allowed the extrapolation of these techniques into other select injury patterns about the hindfoot, and these can be used when dictated by host and injury factors. These situations include ankle fractures as well as midfoot, talus, and calcaneus injuries. Wawrose and colleagues retrospectively evaluated 354 closed ankle-fracture dislocations, of which 28 were selectively placed in a temporizing external fixator and 28 underwent closed reduction, splinting, and discharge from the emergency department.[41] Subsequently, half of the patients in the splint group lost reduction and 5

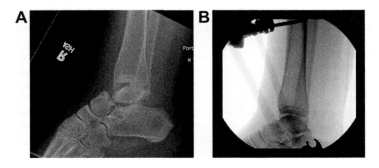

Fig. 3. A polytrauma patient with a talar neck fracture dislocation was unstable for acute ORIF (A). Further, the adjacent soft tissue envelope revealed hemorrhagic fracture blisters. A transfixation pin was applied to the hindfoot for traction, after which a Shantz pin was then inserted percutaneously into the talar body to "joystick" it into a more acceptable alignment. External fixation was then applied as a temporizing measure (B) until definitive ORIF could be performed.

patients (18%) developed anteromedial skin necrosis (Fig. 3). In contrast, no patient in the group undergoing temporizing external fixation was found to have a loss of reduction or skin necrosis; these differences were both statistically significant ($P < .05$). Buyukkuscu and colleagues subsequently confirmed these results in a retrospective study, evaluating splinting versus temporizing external fixation in ankle fracture/dislocations.[42] Similarly, loss of reduction (25%) and soft tissue complications (22%) were significantly higher in the splinting group. In addition, the mean time period between injury and definitive surgery was found to be significantly shorter in the external fixation group compared with the splint group (7 days vs 11 days, respectively). It should also be noted that transarticular Steinmann pins, originally described decades ago,[43] represent an additional option in the armamentarium of staged treatment strategies to impart provisional stability in cases of poor skin conditions or medical issues that preclude early surgery.[19]

OUTCOMES - TEMPORIZING CARE FOR MIDFOOT FRACTURE/DISLOCATIONS

High-energy midfoot injuries, including of the Lisfranc complex, also warrant special attention with respect to soft tissue status before definitive fixation. Kadow and colleagues evaluated 18 polytrauma patients with high-energy midfoot fracture/dislocations who were selectively treated with a staged treatment protocol including external fixation of the midfoot.[44] The authors found that the application of a midfoot spanning external fixator grossly restored midfoot length and alignment in most of the patients, with the loss of acceptable reduction occurring in only one case. No wound complications or deep infections occurred after definitive reconstruction. Subsequently, Arvesen and colleagues reported a series of patients with high-energy midfoot trauma from 2 level I trauma

centers treated in a staged fashion, and detected no significant differences with respect to the length of stay, time to definitive fixation, time to full weight bearing, and return to work whether managed with ORIF or arthrodesis.[45] A separate study by Arvensen and colleagues compared data from 3 level I trauma centers with 29 patients undergoing midfoot external fixation and 15 patients undergoing casting. These data suggested that staged treatment with external fixation led to a delay in the definitive surgical intervention, but was associated with a similar complication rate.[46]

Liu and colleagues retrospectively assessed 21 patients with open Lisfranc fracture/dislocations who underwent a staged progressive reduction technique using a bilateral external fixator over a 4-year period with a mean follow-up of 15.4 months.[47] The mean time to definitive fixation with ORIF or arthrodesis was 18.6 days. Acceptable reductions were achieved and 3 cases of infection, 2 superficial, and 1 deep were managed. By comparison, Herscovici and Scaduto described an alternative approach with the use of 3 or 4 2.0 mm K-wires for the acute stabilization of 18 high-energy Lisfranc dislocations or fracture/dislocations for staged management.[48] These pins were left in situ until definitive fixation was warranted. No patient demonstrated a loss in alignment that was achieved at the time of the index procedure.

OUTCOMES – TEMPORIZING CARE FOR HINDFOOT INJURIES

Temporizing external fixation has also been evaluated in the setting of calcaneus fractures.[49] Farrell and colleagues reported a series of 9 patients with 10 calcaneus fractures who were treated with a protocol of ankle-spanning medial external fixation followed by conversion to a plate via a sinus tarsi approach as the soft tissues allowed.[50] After external fixation, the mean time to definitive fixation was 4.8 days and there were no postoperative wound complications or pin site infections. More recently, Park and colleagues described a damage control strategy in which transarticular pinning was used for staged management of intra-articular calcaneus fractures.[51] In their series, 17 patients with 20 calcaneal fractures were selectively treated with staged management using transarticular K-wires within 24 hours of presentation as a means of restoring calcaneal morphology and stabilizing the soft tissue envelope. The mean Bohler angle increased from $-22°$ to $25°$ after pinning, and conversion to definitive internal fixation occurred at an average of 20 days. No wound complications or infections were reported at a mean 17 months after surgery. Clare and Maloney suggested the use of external fixation in talar neck fracture/dislocations in select cases whereby closed reduction is not possible and provisional stabilization is necessary, after which further advanced imaging can be obtained to facilitate preoperative planning of subsequent semielective care.[52] Mohindra and colleagues also used the use of external fixation after reimplantation of open talar extrusion in 5 cases, with a low rate of deep infection while restoring hindfoot height and preserving options for future reconstruction.[53]

SUMMARY

Severe traumatic foot and ankle injuries may require temporizing procedures due to soft tissue damage, associated injuries, or host-related factors. It is imperative to understand each patient's medical history, injury characteristics, overall injury complex, and medical stability when determining whether to proceed with staged versus definitive care of a traumatic foot or ankle injury. When the decision is made to proceed with a temporizing procedure, several different surgical options have been described, with good outcomes that support their use.

CLINICS CARE POINTS

- Foot and ankle injuries associated with severe concomitant soft tissue trauma should be managed staged
- The work horse for temporizing care is external fixation/closed reduction
- Staged protocols are recommended clinical practice for high energy trauma (ie tibia pilon fracture)

REFERENCES

1. Zelle BA, Dang KH, Ornell SS. High-energy tibial pilon fractures: an instructional review. Int Orthop 2019;43(8):1939–50.
2. McFerran MA, Smith SW, Boulas HJ, et al. Complications encountered in the treatment of pilon fractures. J Orthop Trauma 1992;6(2):195–200.
3. Teeny SM, Wiss DA. Open reduction and internal fixation of tibial plafond fractures. Variables contributing to poor results and complications. Clin Orthop Relat Res 1993;292:108–17.
4. Liporace FA, Yoon RS. Decisions and staging leading to definitive open management of pilon fractures: Where have we come from and where are we now? J Orthop Trauma 2012;26(8):488–98.
5. Fierbinţeanu-Braticevici C, Raspe M, Preda AL, et al. Medical and surgical co-management – A strategy of improving the quality and outcomes of perioperative care. Eur J Intern Med 2019;61: 44–7.
6. Matuszewski PE, Boulton CL, O'Toole RV. Orthopaedic trauma patients and smoking: knowledge deficits and interest in quitting. Injury 2016;47(6): 1206–11.
7. Ernst A, Wilson JM, Ahn J, et al. Malnutrition and the orthopaedic trauma patient: a systematic review of the literature. J Orthop Trauma 2018; 32(10):491–9.
8. Zelle BA, Brown SR, Panzica M, et al. The impact of injuries below the knee joint on the long-term functional outcome following polytrauma. Injury 2005; 36(1):169–77.
9. MacKenzie EJ, Bosse MJ, Pollak AN, et al. Long-term persistence of disability following severe lower-limb trauma. J Bone Joint Surg Am 2005; 87(8):1801–9.
10. Butcher JL, MacKenzie EJ, Cushing B, et al. Long-term outcomes after lower extremity trauma. J Trauma 1996;41(1):4–9.
11. Norris BL, Kellam JF. Soft-tissue injuries associated with high-energy extremity trauma: principles of management. J Am Acad Orthop Surg 1997;5(1): 37–46.
12. Oladeji LO, Platt B, Crist BD. Diabetic pilon fractures: are they as bad as we think? J Orthop Trauma 2021;35(3):149–53.
13. Early JS, Tenenbaum S. Soft tissue management of closed tibial pilon fractures. Tech Orthop 2014; 29(1):2–7.
14. Tosounidis TH, Daskalakis II, Giannoudis PV. Fracture blisters: pathophysiology and management. Injury 2020;51(12):2786–92.
15. Haidukewych GJ. Temporary external fixation for the management of complex intra- and periarticular fractures of the lower extremity. J Orthop Trauma 2002;16(9):678–85.

16. Topliss CJ, Jackson M, Atkins RM. Anatomy of pilon fractures of the distal tibia. J Bone Jt Surg Br 2005;87(5):692–7.

17. Cole PA, Mehrle RK, Bhandari M, et al. The pilon map: fracture lines and comminution zones in OTA/AO type 43C3 pilon fractures. J Orthop Trauma 2013;27(7):e152–6.

18. Englehart MS, Schreiber MA. Measurement of acid-base resuscitation endpoints: Lactate, base deficit, bicarbonate or what? Curr Opin Crit Care 2006; 12(6):569–74.

19. Morgan-Jones RL, Smith KD, Thomas PB. Vertical transtalar Steinmann pin fixation for unstable ankle fractures. Ann R Coll Surg Engl 2000;82(3):185–9.

20. Kapoor SK, Kataria H, Patra SR, et al. Capsuloligamentotaxis and definitive fixation by an ankle-spanning Ilizarov fixator in high-energy pilon fractures. J Bone Jt Surg Br 2010;92(8):1100–6.

21. Lim JA, Thahir A, Zhou AK, et al. Definitive management of open pilon fractures with fine wire fixation. Injury 2020;51(11):2717–22.

22. Anglen JO. Early outcome of hybrid external fixation for fracture of the distal tibia. J Orthop Trauma 1999;13(2):92–7.

23. Pugh KJ, Wolinsky PR, McAndrew MP, et al. Tibial pilon fractures: a comparison of treatment methods. J Trauma 1999;47(5):937–41.

24. Helfet DL, Koval KJ, Pappas J, et al. Intraarticular '"pilon"' fracture of the tibia. Clin Orthop Relat Res 1994;298:221–8.

25. Patterson MJ, Cole JD. Two-staged delayed open reduction and internal fixation of severe pilon fractures. J Orthop Trauma 1999;13(2):85–91.

26. Sirkin M, Sanders R, DiPasquale T, et al. A staged protocol for soft tissue management in the treatment of complex pilon fractures. J Orthop Trauma 1999;13(2):78–84.

27. Wang C, Li Y, Huang L, et al. Comparison of two-staged ORIF and limited internal fixation with external fixator for closed tibial plafond fractures. Arch Orthop Trauma Surg 2010;130(10):1289–97.

28. Tarkin IS, Clare MP, Marcantonio A, et al. An update on the management of high-energy pilon fractures. Injury 2008;39(2):142–54.

29. Swords MP, Weatherford B. High-energy pilon fractures: role of external fixation in acute and definitive treatment. What are the indications and technique for primary ankle arthrodesis? Foot Ankle Clin 2020;25(4):523–36.

30. Barei D, Gardner M, Nork S, et al. Revision of provisional stabilization in pilon fractures referred from outside institutions. Orthop Proc 2011;(93 Supp III): 264–5.

31. Ramlee MH, Abdul Kadir MR, Murali MR, et al. Finite element analysis of three commonly used external fixation devices for treating Type III pilon fractures. Med Eng Phys 2014;36(10):1322–30.

32. Albagli A, Rotman D, Tudor A, et al. Adding a first metatarsal pin to an ankle tubular external fixator does not reduce the incidence of early reduction loss. J Foot Ankle Surg 2021;(21): S1067–2516.

33. Santi MD, Botte MJ. External fixation of the calcaneus and talus: an anatomical study for safe pin insertion. J Orthop Trauma 1996;10(7):487–91.

34. Casey D, McConnell T, Parekh S, et al. Percutaneous pin placement in the medial calcaneus: Is anywhere safe? J Orthop Trauma 2004;18(8 SUPPL):26–9.

35. Shah CM, Babb PE, McAndrew CM, et al. Definitive plates overlapping provisional external fixator pin sites: Is the infection risk increased? J Orthop Trauma 2014;28(9):518–22.

36. Potter JM, van der Vliet QMJ, Esposito JG, et al. Is the proximity of external fixator pins to eventual definitive fixation implants related to the risk of deep infection in the staged management of tibial pilon fractures? Injury 2019;50(11):2103–7.

37. Hadeed MM, Evans CL, Werner BC, et al. Does external fixator pin site distance from definitive implant affect infection rate in pilon fractures? Injury 2019;50(2):503–7.

38. Dombrowsky A, Abyar E, McGwin G, et al. Is definitive plate fixation overlap with external fixator pin sites a risk factor for infection in pilon fractures? J Orthop Trauma 2021;35(1):e7–12.

39. Hardeski D, Gaski G, Joshi M, et al. Can applied external fixators be sterilized for surgery? A prospective cohort study of orthopaedic trauma patients. Injury 2016;47(12):2679–82.

40. Nielsen PJ, Grossman LS, Siebler JC, et al. Is It safe to prep the external fixator in situ during second-stage pilon surgical treatment? J Orthop Trauma 2018;32(3):e102–5.

41. Wawrose RA, Grossman LS, Tagliaferro M, et al. Temporizing external fixation vs splinting following ankle fracture dislocation. Foot Ankle Int 2020;41(2): 177–82.

42. Buyukkuscu MO, Basilgan S, Mollaomeroglu A, et al. Splinting vs temporary external fixation in the initial treatment of ankle fracture-dislocations. Foot Ankle Surg 2021;(21):S1268–7731.

43. Laskin RS. Steinmann-pin fixation in the treatment of unstable fractures of the ankle. J Bone Joint Surg Am 1974;56(3):549–55.

44. Kadow TR, Siska PA, Evans AR, et al. Staged treatment of high energy midfoot fracture dislocations. Foot Ankle Int 2014;35(12):1287–91.

45. Arvesen JE, Burnett Z, Israel H, et al. High-energy midfoot fracture-dislocations: staged treatment with an external fixator. J Surg Orthop Adv 2019; 28(1):24–30.

46. Arvesen J, Burnett Z, Bush AN, et al. High energy midfoot fracture-dislocations: does staged

treatment with external fixation help? J Surg Orthop Adv 2020;29(3):154–8.

47. Liu X, An J, Chen Y, et al. Staged surgical treatment of open lisfranc fracture dislocations using an adjustable bilateral external fixator: A retrospective review of 21 patients. Acta Orthop Traumatol Turc 2020;54(5):488–96.

48. Herscovici D, Scaduto JM. Acute management of high-energy lisfranc injuries: A simple approach. Injury 2018;49(2):420–4.

49. Baumgaertel FR, Gotzen L. Two-stage operative treatment of comminuted os calcis fractures. Primary indirect reduction with medial external fixation and delayed lateral plate fixation. Clin Orthop Relat Res 1993;290:132–41.

50. Farrell BM, Lin CA, Moon CN. Temporising external fixation of calcaneus fractures prior to definitive plate fixation: a case series. Injury 2015;46:S19–22.

51. Park K-H, Oh C-W, Kim J-W, et al. Staged management of severely displaced calcaneal fractures With transarticular pinning: a damage control strategy. Foot Ankle Int 2021. 10711007211013012. online ahead of print.

52. Clare MP, Maloney PJ. Prevention of avascular necrosis with fractures of the talar neck. Foot Ankle Clin 2019;24(1):47–56.

53. Mohindra M, Gogna P, Thora A, et al. Early reimplantation for open total talar extrusion. J Orthop Surg 2014;22(3):304–8.

Spine Section

Severity and Outcome of Neurologic Deficits in Patients with Pyogenic Spondylodiscitis
A Systematic Review

Naveed Nabizadeh, MD[a], Charles H. Crawford III, MD[a,b],
Steven D. Glassman, MD[a,b], John R. Dimar II, MD[a,b],
Leah Y. Carreon, MD, MSc[a,*]

KEYWORDS

- Osteodiscitis • Spondylodiscitis • Vertebral infection • Neurologic impairment
- Neurologic deficit

KEY POINTS

- In certain patients presenting with low back pain, early suspicion of vertebral infection can lead to prompt diagnosis and improved outcomes.
- Higher Frankel grade on presentation may require more aggressive treatment in a timely manner to facilitate neurologic recovery.
- Older age, delayed diagnosis, multilevel involvement, epidural abscess, and more proximal levels of vertebral infection are associated with worse neurologic deficits.

INTRODUCTION

Pyogenic spondylodiscitis is the most common form of hematogenous osteomyelitis in patients older than 50 years and represents 3%–5% of all cases of osteomyelitis.[1] Recently, the incidence of vertebral osteomyelitis has increased because of improved accuracy of diagnosis in addition to the increase in susceptible patients including diabetics, intravenous drug abusers (IVDA), patients undergoing hemodialysis, and immunocompromised hosts.[2]

Neurological symptoms associated with spondylodiscitis have been reported with various patterns, ranging from dysesthesia and radicular pain to complete paraplegia.[3] Previous studies have shown that neurologic deficits develop because of epidural abscesses or a pathologic fracture due to the osteolysis associated with osteomyelitis. Furthermore, the severity of neurologic symptoms is associated with delayed diagnosis, older age, virulence of the offending organism, and the presence of comorbidities.

The purpose of this study is to report on the severity of neurologic impairments associated with spondylodiscitis, response to treatment, and factors contributing to neurologic recovery.

RESEARCH

A comprehensive search of different databases including PubMed, MEDLINE, ScienceDirect,

The manuscript submitted does not contain information about medical devices or drugs. This study reviewed published articles and was determined to be Not Human Subjects Research. Thus, it was exempted from the review by the institutional review board.

[a] Norton Leatherman Spine Center, 210 East Gray Street, Suite 900, Louisville, KY 40202, USA; [b] Department of Orthopaedic Surgery, University of Louisville School of Medicine, 550 South Jackson Street, 1st Floor ACB, Louisville, KY 40202, USA
* Corresponding author.
E-mail address: Leah.Carreon@nortonhealthcare.org

and Google Scholar from 2000 to 2020 was performed. The searched keywords included "Vertebral Osteomyelitis" OR "Osteodiscitis" OR "Pyogenic Spondylodiscitis" AND "Neurologic Impairment" OR "Neurologic Deficit." Manual search of reference lists from relevant articles and guidelines was performed.

Initially, 1478 articles were collected and their abstracts were screened. Seventy-five articles were selected based on inclusion and exclusion criteria. After comprehensive review of full texts, 40 studies that contained detailed neurologic examinations were eligible for inclusion in this systematic review (Table 1).

Study Selection Criteria
The inclusion criteria were as follows: (1) studies on adult patients with confirmed pyogenic spondylodiscitis, treated conservatively or surgically, (2) studies that reported objective neurologic examinations before and after an appropriate treatment, and (3) studies published in English. Studies on nonpyogenic spondylodiscitis, animal studies, studies on iatrogenic infections, and articles lacking specific description of neurologic findings were excluded.

Data extraction
The extracted data from each study consisted of the number of cases with neurologic symptoms, mean age, gender distribution, location of involved levels, time period before appropriate treatment was instituted, epidural abscess, neurologic status at initial presentation, and the last follow-up visit.

Data Analysis
All statistical analyses were performed using IBM SPSS Statistics for Windows, version 27.0 (Armonk, NY). Pooling of data within subgroups was performed using weighted averages based on the sample size. Categorical variables were assessed using the Fischer exact test. A P value less than .05 was considered statistically significant.

Classification of Neurologic Manifestations and Sequelae
The neurologic status was reported using different definitions. However, the most commonly used classification for neurologic deficits was Frankel grading[42] which is similar to International Standards for the Neurological Classification of Spinal Cord Injury (ISNCSCI) designed by the American Spinal Injury Association (ASIA) (Box 1).[43]

We proposed certain equivalents for the Frankel grading to categorize the reported neurologic status. Conditions described as "severe or marked," "paraplegic or tetraplegic or quadriplegic," "paralysis," "complete cord," "myelopathy," and "cauda equina" were considered equivalent to Frankel grades A and B. The reported physical examinations did not allow us to easily distinguish between grade A and grade B. The neurologic manifestations described as "moderate," "paresis," "foot drop," and "incomplete cord" were taken into account as Frankel grade C. Reported symptoms such as "mild," "minimal," and "subjective" weakness were assumed equal to Frankel grade D. The "pure sensory problems," "only numbness," "radicular pain," and "sciatalgia" were categorized as Frankel grade E. The neurologic results of treatment, medically or surgically, were divided into complete recovery (regain normal sensory and motor functions), partial recovery (1- or 2-grade improvement in the motor functions), unchanged, and deterioration (worsening of neurologic status).

RESULTS
Study Characteristics and Limitation
Almost all the authors assessed the neurologic outcomes retrospectively. Thus, the bias and limitations, relevant to retrospective studies, are carried into this systematic review.

Demographic Data
Three thousand two hundred thirty-six patients with pyogenic spondylodiscitis were included with a mean age of 60.3 years. There were 1966 males (62%) out of 3162 reporting gender data. Delay in treatment, by a mean of 56.24 days, was discovered in 1828 cases with symptoms of vertebral infection.

In addition, there was multilevel involvement in 513 (16%) of 3212 patients. The most common location of vertebral infection was the lumbar and thoracolumbar spine (60%), followed by the thoracic spine (27%) and then the cervical spine (13%). The incidence of neurologic deficit concomitant with epidural abscess was 53% (1228 out of 2331). The studies that focused only on cervical spondylodiscitis demonstrated a higher risk of neurologic symptoms (52%, 37 of 71 cases) and greater frequency of epidural abscess formation (72%, 36 of 50 cases) than the studies focused on noncervical involvements.

Neurologic Manifestations and Sequelae
Among 3236 spondylodiscitis cases, 1314 patients had a variety of neurologic manifestations: 415 (32%) presented with subjective symptoms including radicular pain, sciatica, or numbness,

Table 1 Contributing studies						
Study	Sample Size	Significant Neurologic Deficit	Surgical Approach	Neurologic Deficit Improved	Neurologic Deficit Unchanged	Epidural Abscess
Asamoto & Doi,[4] 2005	27	16	17	22	4	17
Ascione & Balato,[5] 2017	30	5	0	18	4	—
Bernard & Dinh,[6] 2015	359	19	0	47	10	—
Bettini & Girardo,[7] 2009	56	5	8	3	2	3
Cervan & de Dios Colmenero,[8] 2012	23	12	7	5	7	14
Chin-Pea & Ma,[9] 2012	48	28	48	28	0	35
Dimar et al,[10] 2004	42	3	42	3	0	1
Dragsted & Aagaard,[11] 2017	65	23	65	12	6	46
Kim & Melikian,[12] 2014	127	40	20	14	6	355
Elsaid & Makhlouf,[13] 2015	19	15	19	11	2	15
Erick & Flipo,[14] 2001	110	18	0	18	0	—
Gupta & Kowalski,[3] 2014	260	42	127	35	7	158
Hadjpavlou et al,[15] 2000	101	17	58	8	9	39
Heyde et al,[16] 2006	20	8	19	8	0	12
Karadimas et al,[17] 2008	163	22	93	5	4	—
Lee & Kim,[18] 2018	51	36	29	32	4	28
Livorsi & Daver,[19] 2008	35	8	9	2	6	26
McHenry et al,[20] 2002	253	48	109	33	15	43
Masuda & Miyamoto,[21] 2006	5	5	5	3	2	2
Matsubara & Yamada,[22] 2018	52	22	21	9	3	30
Mavrogenis & Igoumenou,[23] 2016	153	11	13	10	1	5
Nolla et al,[24] 2002	64	18	4	16	2	39
Ozkan & Wrede,[25] 2014	21	17	21	11	4	—
Robach & Niethammer,[26] 2014	135	33	75	23	10	46
Rosinsky & Mandler,[27] 2018	16	8	15	7	1	2
Schinkel & Gottwald,[28] 2003	32	17	32	7	7	19
Schuster & Anthony,[29] 2000	47	13	47	8	5	33
Shiban & Janssen,[30] 2014	113	40	113	36	2	33
Shiban & Janssen,[31] 2014	25	7	25	4	3	11
Shousha & Boehm,[32] 2012	30	12	30	7	0	24
Siddiq et al,[33] 2004	57	33	28	5	8	57
Sobottke et al,[34] 2010	32	8	16	5	2	12
Curry & Hoh,[35] 2005	48	27	25	12	9	48
Urrutia et al,[36] 2013	102	44	16	44	0	11

(continued on next page)

Study	Sample Size	Significant Neurologic Deficit	Surgical Approach	Neurologic Deficit Improved	Neurologic Deficit Unchanged	Epidural Abscess
Valacius & Hansen,[37] 2013	196	14	105	8	6	60
Woergen et al,[38] 2006	62	15	34	8	7	8
Yoshimoto et al,[39] 2011	45	26	15	23	3	—
Zarrouk et al,[40] 2007	29	15	7	9	6	19
Dennis et al,[41] 2017	84	39	19	19	0	—

whereas 899 cases (68%) had a significant neurologic deficit defined as Frankel grades A, B, C, or D (Table 2).

Although the Frankel grades A and B, the most severe subtypes of neurologic deficits, constituted a smaller group (22%) of patients,

---

Box 1
International Standards for the Neurological Classification of Spinal Cord Injury (ISNCSCI) designed by the ASIA

A = Complete.

There is no motor function or sensation. No motor or sensation was preserved in sacral segments S4–5.

B = Sensory incomplete.

Sensory but not motor function is preserved less than the neurologic level and includes the sacral segments S4–5 (light touch or pinprick at S4–5 or deep anal pressure), and no motor function is preserved more than 3 levels less than the motor level on either side of the body.

C = Motor incomplete.

Motor function is preserved less than the neurologic level, and more than half of the key muscles less than the injury level have a muscle grade less than 3.

D = Motor incomplete.

Motor function is preserved less than the neurologic level, and at least half of the key muscle functions below the injury level have a muscle grade of at least 3 or higher.

E = Normal

Once sensation and motor function are graded as normal in all segments in a person with prior deficits, they are given an American Spine Injury Association (ASIA) of E. A person without an initial spinal cord injury does not receive an ASIA grade.

they had the lowest rate of complete recovery (16%, $P<.001$) and the highest rate of remaining unchanged after treatment (34%).

Among Frankel grade C cases (n = 333), 53% achieved partial recovery whereas 29% obtained complete recovery. In patients with Frankel grade D (n = 280), more than half had complete recovery (53%) whereas a quarter of patients sustained partial (25%) or no recovery (20%). About 50% (n = 449) of cases with significant neurologic symptoms promptly underwent surgery after the confirmation of diagnosis, whereas 353 patients (39%) underwent surgical intervention between 1 and 14 months after diagnosis and medical treatment failure.

We compared the outcome of neurologic impairment in the patients who were treated nonsurgically (n = 97) with the patients who underwent surgical procedure initially (n = 449). Surgical intervention was associated with a higher rate of neurologic recovery (R = − 0.205, $P<.000$).

DISCUSSION

The current study highlights the relatively poor prognosis of neurologic deficits associated with pyogenic spondylodiscitis. Delays in diagnosis and treatment can lead to progressive infection that spreads into the spinal canal resulting in epidural abscess formation.[44,45] The compressive effects of epidural abscesses cause severe pain in addition to myelopathy and radiculopathy.[46] In addition, associated ischemia and infarction of the spinal cord can aggravate the neurologic status. Furthermore, vertebral bone destruction (osteolysis) and secondary spinal instability potentially exacerbate canal compromise.[47]

The rate of neurologic compromise has been reported from 7% by Hadjipavlou up to 57% by Curry Jr and colleagues. At least a simple extremity weakness manifests in 79% of patients with neurologic impairment.[8,15,35,48] Petkova

Table 2
Neurologic recovery stratified by Frankel grade

Frankel Grade	Complete Recovery	Partial Recovery	Unchanged	Deteriorated	Total
Frankel grades A and B	45 (16%)	137 (48%)	98 (34%)	6 (2%)	286 (22%)
Frankel grade C	97 (29%)	178 (53%)	53 (16%)	5 (2%)	333 (25%)
Frankel grade D	149 (53%)	71 (25%)	55 (20%)	5 (2%)	280 (21%)
Total	291 (32%)	386 (43%)	206 (23%)	16 (2%)	899

and colleagues reported neurologic symptoms in one-third of the cases and ranged from radicular pain to radiculopathy (29%) to paresis (2%–13%) and cauda equina syndrome (10%).[49] Current systematic review demonstrated radicular pain and absence of motor deficit in 32% of patients. However, in this current review, motor deficits were reported in 68% of patients which consisted of 22% Frankel grades A & B, 25% Frankel grade C, and 21% Frankel grade D.

The high frequency of Frankel grade A and B cases, those presenting with paraplegia or cauda equina syndrome, might be attributed to age, delayed diagnosis, epidural abscess formation, multilevel involvement, or cord level involvement. The role of these factors in the development of neurologic impairment was assessed:

1. Age: In the past decades, the most frequently affected people were elderly patients who more often experience multiple comorbidities and are infected with drug-resistant organisms, particularly Methicillin Resistant S. aureus (MRSA).[46] However, the current study demonstrated a shift of neurologic symptoms to the younger ages (range: 43–70 years, median: 60.3 years), which is likely attributed to the increased number of IVDAs.
2. Delayed diagnosis: The delayed diagnosis of spondylodiscitis, reported between 1 and 6 months, has a significant impact on the natural history and the neurologic outcome.[48,49] This systematic review demonstrated delayed diagnosis in patients with spondylodiscitis, roughly 56.2 days (from 10 to 120 days), and also confirmed its association with a higher risk of neurologic deficit.
3. Epidural abscesses formation: Epidural abscess has been commonly reported in patients with significant neurologic deficits, leading to myelopathy, radiculopathy, or back pain.[15] Recent review showed that epidural abscess occurs in 56% of

spondylodiscitis cases who present with neurologic symptoms.
4. Multilevel involvement: Vertebral osteomyelitis has been discovered mostly in the lumbar, then thoracic, and then cervical levels. Multilevel involvement has been reported in 3% to 13% of patients.[15,50] We found the distribution of spinal infection resembling the previous studies and the likelihood of multilevel involvement in the patients with neurologic deficits was approximately 16%. Presumably, multiple episodes of sepsis, particularly in IVDAs, can explain the frequency of multilevel spondylodiscitis associated with neurologic involvement.
5. Cord level involvement: This review confirmed that cervical level involvement predisposes the patient to a higher risk of neurologic impairment. We discovered neurologic deficits in 52% and epidural abscess in 72% of cervical spondylodiscitis cases.

Conventional treatment of spondylodiscitis involves antibiotic therapy for 6 to 12 weeks with surgical intervention reserved for the circumstances with failure of medical management.[44,48,51] However, great diligence must be maintained during conservative treatment because the rapid progression of bony destruction, instability, segmental kyphosis, and neurologic deficit will demand the addition of prompt surgical treatment. Neurologic compromise has convinced authors to suggest different treatments. Yoshimoto and colleagues evaluated the results of conservative treatment in paralyzed patients who were not able to undergo surgery because of poor general condition. He discovered that paralysis improved in 73% of these patients with nonoperative treatment.[39] Cheung and colleagues believe that only 10% to 20% of patients suffering from pyogenic spondylitis require open surgery. He also expressed that surgical decompression could improve the prognosis of neurologic recovery much better than nonoperative management.[52] Graeff and colleagues pointed out that epidural abscess, multilevel osteomyelitis, or diabetes escalate the risk of failure of conservative treatment.[53] McHenry concluded that surgical intervention in the patients with neurologic compromise brings about a favorable outcome in nearly 70% and even better results were achieved in the absence of diagnostic delay.[20] Zarghooni and colleagues reported persisted motor deficit in 30% and hypoesthesia in 90% after surgical approach but the quality of life and patients' satisfaction were higher in the surgically treated group.[54] Lerner and colleagues identified an improvement of neurologic deficits after surgery in 76% of cases, whereas 20% showed few changes. Hadjipavlou and colleagues demonstrated that only 23% of patients with paralysis on admission recovered completely after surgical decompression.[15]

We compared the frequency and outcome of treatment in different Frankel groups. Approximately 11% of circumstances with deficits responded to medical treatment, whereas 39% underwent surgical approach from 1 to 14 months after diagnosis because of the resistance or recurrence of symptoms. Furthermore, 50% of patients required prompt surgery because of severe (Frankel grade A or B) or progressive neurologic impairment.

Frankel groups A, B, and C with significant impairment sustained complete recovery only in 16% and 29% of cases. Nevertheless, unhesitating and appropriate treatment provided partial recovery or at least halted the progression of neurologic compromise in about 82% and 69% of circumstances, respectively. Regardless of the severity and the type of treatment, the neurologic status deteriorated in about 2% of cases.

SUMMARY

Considering the remarkable number of severe neurologic deficits in addition to their poor recovery even after surgical intervention, it is crucial to establish the diagnosis and start appropriate treatment of pyogenic spondylodiscitis in a timely manner. Surgical treatment is associated with a higher rate of neurologic recovery in patients with pyogenic spondylodiscitis presenting with neurologic deficit. The results of this systematic review can help clinicians better understand prognosis and thereby improve patient counseling and informed consent processes.

CLINICS CARE POINTS

- Pyogenic spondylodiscitis can present with neurologic deficits because of abscess formation, pathologic fracture, kyphotic deformity, or neural ischemia.
- Delayed diagnosis, older age, virulent organism, comorbidities, and multilevel involvement increase the risk of neurologic deficit.
- More severe neurologic deficits on presentation are associated with less recovery and worse outcomes.
- Surgical treatment is associated with a higher rate of neurologic recovery.
- Spinal instability, epidural abscess, and progressive neurologic deficit are indications for prompt surgical treatment.

DISCLOSURE

The authors have nothing to disclose.

REFERENCES

1. Jensen AG, Espersen F, Skinhøj P, et al. Increasing frequency of vertebral osteomyelitis following Staphylococcus aureus bacteraemia in Denmark 1980-1990. J Infect 1997;34(2):113–8.
2. Duarte RM, Vaccaro AR. Spinal infection: state of the art and management algorithm. Eur Spine J 2013;22:2787–99.
3. Gupta A, Kowalski TJ. Long-term outcome of pyogenic vertebral osteomyelitis: a cohort study of 260 patients. Open Forum Infect Dis 2014;1(3):ofu107.
4. Asamoto S, Doi H. Spondylodiscitis: diagnosis and treatment. Surg Neurol 2005;64:103–8.
5. Ascione T, Balato G. Clinical and microbiological outcomes in haematogenous spondylodiscitis treated conservatively. Eur Spine J 2017;26(Suppl 4):S489–95.
6. Bernard L, Dinh A. Antibiotic treatment for 6 weeks versus 12 weeks in patients with pyogenic vertebral osteomyelitis: an open-label, non-inferiority, randomized, controlled trial. Lancet 2015; 385:875–82.
7. Bettini N, Girardo M. Evaluation of conservative treatment of non specific Spondylodiscitis. Eur Spine J 2009;18(Suppl 1):S143–50.
8. Cervan AM, de Dios Colmenero J. Spondylodiscitis in patients under haemodyalisis. Int Orthop 2012; 36:421–6.

9. Lin CP, Ma HL. Surgical results of long posterior fixation with short fusion in the treatment of pyogenic spondylodiscitis of the thoracic and lumbar spine. Spine 2012;37(25):E1572–9.

10. Dimar JR, Carreon LY, Glassman SD, et al. Treatment of pyogenic vertebral osteomyelitis with anterior debridement and fusion followed by delayed posterior spinal fusion. Spine 2004;29(3):326–32.

11. Dragsted C, Aagaard T. Mortality and health-related quality of life in patients surgically treated for spondylodiscitis. J Orthop Surg 2017;25(2):1–8.

12. Kim SD, Melikian R. Independent predictors of failure of nonoperative management of spinal epidural abscesses. Spine J 2014;14:1673–9.

13. Ahmed E, Makhlouf M. Surgical management of spontaneous pyogenic spondylodiscitis: clinical and radiological outcome. Egypt J Neurosurg 2015;30(3):221–6.

14. Legrand E, Flipo RM. Management of nontuberculous infectious discitis. Treatments used in 110 patients admitted to 12 teaching hospitals in France. Joint Bone Spine 2001;68:504–9.

15. Hadjipavlou AG, Mader JT, Necessary JT, et al. Hematogenous pyogenic spinal infections and their surgical management. Spine 2000;25:1668–79.

16. Heyde CE, Boehm H, El Saghir H, et al. Surgical treatment of spondylodiscitis in the cervical spine: aminimum 2-year follow-up. Eur Spine J 2006;15:1380–7.

17. Karadimas EJ, Bunger C, Lindblad BE, et al. Spondylodiscitis. A retrospective study of 163 patients. Acta Orthop 2008;79:650–9.

18. Lee Y, Kim BJ. Comparative analysis of spontaneous infectious spondylitis: pyogenic versus tuberculous. J Korean Neurosurg Soc 2018;61(1):81–8.

19. Livorsi DJ, Daver NG. Outcomes of treatment for hematogenous Staphylococcus aureus vertebral osteomyelitis in the MRSA ERA. J Infect 2008;57:128e131.

20. McHenry MC, Easly KA, Locker GA. Vertebral osteomyelitis:long-term outcome for 253 patients from 7 Cleveland-area hospitals. Clin Infect Dis 2002;34:1342–50.

21. Masuda T, Miyamoto K. Surgical treatment with spinal instrumentation for pyogenic spondylodiscitis due to methicillin-resistant Staphylococcus aureus(MRSA): a report of five cases. Arch Orthop Trauma Surg 2006;126:339–45.

22. Matsubara T, Yamada K. Clinical outcomes of percutaneous suction aspiration and drainage for the treatment of infective spondylodiscitis with paravertebral or epidural abscess. Spine J 2018;18:1558–69.

23. Mavrogenis AF, Igoumenou V. When and how to operate on spondylodiscitis: a report of 13 patients. Eur J Orthop Surg Traumatol 2016;26:31–40.

24. Nolla JM, Ariza J, Gómez-Vaquero C, et al. Spontaneous pyogenic vertebral osteomyelitis in nondrug users. Semin Arthritis Rheum 2002;31:271–8.

25. Özkan N, Wrede K. Cervical spondylodiscitis – A clinical analysis of surgically treated patients and review of the literature. Clin Neurol Neurosurg 2014;117:86–92.

26. Robbach BP, Niethammer TR. Surgical treatment of patients with spondylodiscitis and neurological deficits caused by Spinal Epidural Abscess (SEA) is a predictor of clinical outcome. J Spinal Disord Tech 2014;27:395–400.

27. Rosinsky P, Mandler S. Antibiotic-resistant spondylodiscitis with canal invasion and aggressive evolution to epidural abscess: a case series of spontaneous occurrence in 16 patients. Int J Spine Surg 2018;12(6):743–50.

28. Schinkel C, Gottwald M. Surgical treatment of spondylodiscitis. Surg Infect 2003;4(4):387–91.

29. Schuster JM, Anthony M. Use of structural allografts in spinal osteomyelitis: a review of 47 cases. J Neurosurg 2000;93:8–14.

30. Shiban E, Janssen I. A retrospective study of 113 consecutive cases of surgically treated spondylodiscitis patients. A single-center experience. Acta Neurochir 2014;156:1189–96.

31. Shiban E, Janssen I. Spondylodiscitis by drug- multiresistant bacteria: a single-center experience of 25 cases. Spine J 2014;14:2826–34.

32. Shousha M, Boehm H. Surgical treatment of cervical spondylodiscitis. A review of 30 consecutive patients. Spine 2012;37(1):E30–6.

33. Siddiq F, Chowfin A, Tight R, et al. Medical vs surgical management of spinal epidural abscess. Arch Intern Med 2004;164:2409–12.

34. Sobottke R, Röllinghoff M, Zarghooni K, et al. Spondylodiscitis in the elderly patient: clinical mid-term results and quality of life. Arch Orthop Trauma Surg 2010;130:1083–91.

35. Curry WT, Hoh BL. Spinal epidural abscess: clinical presentation, management, and outcome. Surg Neurol 2005;63:364–71.

36. Urrutia J, Campos M, Zamora T, et al. Doe's pathogen identification influence clinical outcomes in patients with pyogenic spinal infections? J Spinal Disord Tech 2013.

37. Valancius K, Hansen ES. Failure modes in conservative and surgical managementof infectious spondylodiscitis. Eur Spine J 2013;22:1837–44.

38. Woertgen C, Rothoerl RD, Englert C, et al. Pyogenic spinal infections and outcome according to the 36-item short form health survey. J Neurosurg Spine 2006;4:441–6.

39. Yoshimoto M, Takebayashi T, Kawaguchi S, et al. Pyogenic spondylitis in the elderly: a report from Japan with the most aging society. Eur Spine J 2011;20(4):649–54.

40. Zarrouk V, Feydy A, Sallés F, et al. Imaging does not predict the clinical outcome of bacterial vertebral osteomyelitis. Rheumatology 2007;46(2):292–5.

41. Dennis Hey HW, Nathaniel Ng LW, Tan CS, et al. Spinal implants can be inserted in patients with deep spine infection— results from a large cohort study. Spine (Phila Pa 1976) 2017;42(8):E490–5.

42. Frankel HL, Hancock DO, Hyslop G, et al. The value of postural reduction in initial management of closed injuries of the spine with paraplegia and tetraplegia, I. Paraplegia 1969;7:179–1192.

43. Kirshblum SC, Biering-Sørensen F, Betz R, et al. International standards for neurological classification of spinal cord injury: cases with classification challenges. Top Spinal Cord Inj Rehabil 2014;20(2):81–9.

44. Herren C, Jung N. Spondylodiscitis: diagnosis and treatment options. A systematic review. Dtsch Arztebl Int 2017;114(51-52):875.

45. Cornett CA, Vincent SA. Bacterial Spine infections in adults: evaluation and management. J Am Acad Orthop Surg 2016;24(1):11–8.

46. Fantoni M, Trecarichi EM, Rossi B, et al. Epidemiological and clinical features of pyogenic spondylodiscitis. Eur Rev Med Pharmacol Sci 2012;16(Suppl 2):2–7.

47. Babinchak TJ, Riley DK, Rotheram EB Jr. Pyogenic vertebral osteomyelitis of the posterior elements. Clin Infect Dis 1997;25:221–4.

48. Butler JS, Shelly MJ, Timlin M, et al. Non tuberculous pyogenic spinal infection in adults: a 12-year experience from a tertiary referral center. Spine 2006;31:2695–700.

49. Petkova1 AS, Zhelyazkov1 CB. Spontaneous spondylodiscitis - epidemiology, clinical features, diagnosis and treatment. Folia Med (Plovdiv) 2017; 59(3):254–60.

50. Mylona E, Samarkos M, Kakalou E, et al. Pyogenic vertebral osteomyelitis: a systematic review of clinical characteristics. Semin Arthritis Rheum 2009;39: 10–7.

51. Ahmed A, Jahangira N. Management of Pyogenic Spinal Infection, review of literature. J Orthopaedics 2019;16:508–12.

52. Cheung WY, Keith DK. Pyogenic spondylitis. Int Orthop 2012;36:397–404.

53. de Graeff JJ, Pereira NR, van Wulfften Palthe OD, et al. Prognostic factors for failure of antibiotic treatment in patients with osteomyelitis of the spine. Spine (Phila Pa 1976) 2017;42:1339–46.

54. Zarghooni K, Röllinghoff M, Sobottke R, et al. Treatment of spondylodiscitis. Int Orthop 2012;36: 405–11.

Postoperative Epidural Hematoma

Mladen Djurasovic, MD*, Chad Campion, MD, John R. Dimar II, MD,
Steven D. Glassman, MD, Jeffrey L. Gum, MD

KEYWORDS

- Postoperative epidural hematoma • Risk factors • Anticoagulation • Drain • Complication

---

KEY POINTS

- A symptomatic postoperative epidural hematoma is a rare complication of spine surgery but can lead to permanent neurologic deficits and severe long-term disability.
- Risk factors for epidural hematoma include age, preoperative or postoperative anticoagulation, or multilevel laminectomy.
- When epidural hematoma is suspected, an emergent MRI should be obtained and surgical evacuation of the hematoma should be done as quickly as possible.

INTRODUCTION

Postoperative epidural hematoma is a rare but potentially devastating complication of spine surgery. As the rate of spine procedures continues to rise in the United States,[1] there has been a stakeholder driven movement toward value-based health care, with a focus on health-related quality of life, patient reported outcomes, and the avoidance of complications. In spine surgery, many perioperative complications such as incidental durotomy or urinary tract infections will have only temporary effects on patient outcomes.[2] However other complications, such as epidural hematoma, can lead to severe impairment and permanent disability. A symptomatic epidural hematoma is an accumulation of blood in the spinal canal which compresses the thecal sac, cauda equina, or spinal cord, leading to neurologic dysfunction. Although surgery is the most common cause, it can happen spontaneously, from trauma, from anticoagulation, with bleeding from spinal cord vascular anomalies (eg, AVM), from epidural steroid injections or from spinal or epidural anesthesia.[3] The purpose of this article is to review the epidemiology, etiology, diagnosis, and treatment of symptomatic postoperative epidural hematoma.

Epidural hematomas should be a focus for all spine surgeons, given the potentially catastrophic long-term effects. A high index of suspicion and prompt recognition and treatment is critical in maximizing patient outcome.[4]

INCIDENCE AND EPIDEMIOLOGY

Symptomatic epidural hematoma following spine surgery is rare, with multiple large case series reporting an incidence of less than 1%.[5] A distinction must be made between symptomatic and asymptomatic postoperative epidural hematomas, as *asymptomatic* epidural hematoma is extremely common following lumbar surgery. Mirzai[6] performed a randomized controlled trial of subfascial drain use following lumbar discectomy. He studied all patients with an MRI on postoperative day 1 and found 89% had a radiographic epidural hematoma. None of these patients exhibited symptoms. Similarly, Sokolowski[7] found that in a prospective study of 50 patients undergoing laminectomy, 58% had MRI evidence of an asymptomatic epidural hematoma. Many patients who require an MRI for some reason in the early postoperative period will have evidence of epidural hematoma on MRI without exhibiting symptoms. Thus, it

---

Norton Leatherman Spine Center, 210 East Gray Street, #900, Louisville, KY 40202, USA
* Corresponding Author:
E-mail address: djuraso@hotmail.com

Orthop Clin N Am 53 (2022) 113–121
https://doi.org/10.1016/j.ocl.2021.08.006
0030-5898/22/

seems that asymptomatic epidural hematomas are much more common than symptomatic epidural hematomas. Why some progress to become symptomatic is unknown but is likely multifactorial, depending on the pressure generated by the fluid, specific aspects of patient's anatomy, intrinsic reserve of the patient's neurologic structures, extent of the surgical decompression, as well as other factors.

Several large retrospective case series have reported an overall incidence of symptomatic postoperative epidural hematoma between 0.10% and 0.69%.[8–17] These series are summarized in Table 1. These data again generally represent the incidence of *symptomatic* postoperative epidural hematoma requiring return to surgery.

Several of these case series have included an analysis of risk factors for development of symptomatic hematoma, but the results have varied between studies. Awad and colleagues[10] reviewed nearly 15,000 consecutive cases at Johns Hopkins and found an overall incidence of 0.20% for symptomatic epidural hematoma. He identified preoperative, intraoperative, and postoperative risk factors. Preoperative risk factors included NSAID use, Rh-positive blood type, and age greater than 60. Intraoperative risk factors included surgeries greater than 5 levels, blood loss greater than 1L, and hemoglobin less than 10 g/dL. Postoperative, he identified Coumadin use as a risk factor when the INR was allowed to exceed 2.0 in the first 24 hours after surgery. Kou and colleagues[8] reviewed the single-center experience with epidural hematoma at Beaumont over a 10-year period. Using a case-control study design, the authors found that multilevel procedures and preoperative coagulopathy were significant risk factors, but that age, body mass, and drain use were not. Studies from Japan suggest that poorly controlled hypertension in the perioperative period may also contribute to epidural hematoma.[18,19] Many of the reported studies in the literature have the common limitation that the incidence of symptomatic epidural hematoma is so rare that statistical power to study risk factors is limited by the low numbers of cases. Knusel and colleagues[15] report the largest series in the literature which is a database study of the National Surgical Quality Improvement Program (NSQIP) database. They identified age, obesity, perioperative transfusion, multilevel surgery, dural repair, and microscope use as independent risk factors for reoperation for epidural hematoma. However, their analysis was limited in that it could only include those variables which were measured and recorded

in the NSQIP database. Overall, looking at the literature as a whole, age, multilevel procedures, and preoperative or postoperative coagulopathy were found to be risk factors in multiple studies, but the issue of what predisposes a given patient to developing a clinically important epidural hematoma remains an issue requiring further study.

SURGICAL PATHOPHYSIOLOGY

A symptomatic epidural hematoma develops postoperatively when the neural elements have been uncovered by a decompressive procedure (laminectomy or laminotomy), and then continued bleeding in the confined subfascial space leads to build up of blood under pressure, and subsequent mechanical compression of the neural elements and neurologic dysfunction. Continued bleeding beneath the fascia can arise from multiple sources, including epidural veins, muscle surfaces, and bone surfaces which have been decorticated as part of a fusion procedure. Batson's plexus is a rich network of veins found throughout the epidural space and can bleed quite briskly, particularly with posterior interbody fusion procedures. This plexus is partially decompressed by operative positioning with the abdomen dependent on a spine dedicated table, but sometimes this can be challenging in patients with obesity and epidural veins can bleed quite briskly. In addition, small arterial vessels are typically present lateral to the facet joints and pars interarticularis and can be injured during exposure of the transverse processes during a posterolateral fusion procedure. Small arteries and veins in the paraspinal musculature are often injured during exposure but may be suppressed by self-retaining retractors and may become active again after removal of retractors at the conclusion of the procedure. Hemostasis should always be carefully achieved at all points during the surgical procedure using numerous available hemostatic agents and bipolar electrocautery and should be critically assessed at the conclusion of the procedure before closure. Dealing with a significant bleeding source at this point during the initial surgical procedure is certainly preferable to returning a patient to the OR when a hematoma causes symptoms.

ROLE OF PHARMACOLOGIC ANTICOAGULATION AFTER SPINAL SURGERY

The role of pharmacologic anticoagulation after elective spine surgery is an area of some current

Table 1
Incidence of symptomatic epidural hematoma in large retrospective case series

Reference	Study type	Number of cases analyzed	Number of symptomatic epidural hematomas	Incidence (%)
Kou et al,[8] 2002	Retrospective, single center	12,000	12	0.10%
Uribe et al,[9] 2003	Retrospective, single center	4018	9	0.22%
Awad et al,[10] 2005	Retrospective, single center	14,932	32	0.21%
Yi et al,[11] 2006	Retrospective, single center	3720	9	0.24%
Aono et al,[12] 2011	Retrospective, single center	6356	26	0.41%
Amiri et al,[13] 2013	Retrospective, multicenter	4568	10	0.22%
Kao et al,[14] 2015	Retrospective, single center	15,562	25	0.16%
Knusel et al,[15] 2020	NSQIP database	75,878	206	0.27%
Masuda et al,[16] 2020	Retrospective, multicenter	10,680	45	0.4%
Hohenberger et al,[17] 2020	Retrospective, single center	6024	42	0.69%

controversy, and its effect on the incidence of postoperative epidural hematomas is unknown. Generally speaking, both deep venous thrombosis (DVT) and pulmonary embolism (PE) are much less common following spinal surgery than other orthopedic procedures such as total knee or total hip replacement.[20] Fineberg and colleagues[21] performed an NSQIP database study and found the overall risk for DVT following elective lumbar spine surgery was only 0.34%, and the risk of PE was 0.18%. A limitation of this study is that incidence rates represent only those cases that were actively worked up, diagnosed, and thus reflected in the medical record and NSQIP database. It did not include undetected thromboembolic disease. Cheng[22] performed a systematic review of the literature and found that in the absence of chemoprophylaxis, the risk of a thromboembolic complication following elective spine surgery is about 2.3% for degenerative lumbar surgery and about 5.3% for thoracolumbar deformity surgery. Given these low rates of thromboembolic disease, most centers focus on early postoperative mobilization and ambulation of patients and the use of sequential compressive devices in order to prevent DVT's following spine surgery. Pharmacologic prophylaxis generally has been

avoided because of the perceived risk of developing a compressive epidural hematoma. For patients who require preoperative anticoagulation for chronic medical conditions (eg, atrial fibrillation, mechanical heart valve, or a history of PE), chemoprophylaxis is usually resumed 48 to 72 hours following surgery, often in consultation with the patient's medical team. However, there are no clear guidelines regarding when it is safe to resume anticoagulation following spine surgery.

Despite the relatively low rates of thromboembolic disease following elective spine surgery, some centers are trying to lower rates further by using routine pharmacologic prophylaxis.[23] The incidence of epidural hematoma in these reports has generally been low, but a common limitation of these studies is that they are generally underpowered to detect changes in incidence of postoperative hematomas. Cox[24] performed a retrospective cohort study, where they compared a series of patients who received SCD's along with 5000 IU of unfractionated subcutaneous heparin, to a historical cohort who used SCD's only. The rate of DVT was statistically significantly lowered from 2.7% to 1.0%, with no change in PE rate. The rate of epidural hematoma was 0.6% in the nonprophylaxis group (n = 944) and 0.4% in the heparin group (n = 992), with no significant difference between groups. Gerlach[25] reported a retrospective case series of 1954 elective surgery patients treated with low-molecular-weight heparin (nadroparin) within 24 hours after surgery. Thirteen patients (0.7%) developed postoperative epidural hematoma, with most diagnosed before the administration of LMWH. Similarly, Voth[26] and Schizas[27] used an LMWH protocol in postoperative patients and reported symptomatic epidural hematoma rates of 0% and 0.7%, respectively. Rokito and colleagues[28] performed a prospective study comparing thromboembolic deterrent (TED) stockings (n = 42), TED stockings with SCD's (n = 33), and TED stockings with postoperative coumadin (n = 35). No DVT's, PE's, or epidural hematomas were detected. In summary, multiple studies which have looked at the use of pharmacologic prophylaxis after routine spine surgery have reported symptomatic epidural hematoma rates of less than 1%. However, no clear guidelines have been developed regarding the need for chemoprophylaxis after routine elective spine surgery, and this remains an area of some debate.

ROLE OF POSTOPERATIVE WOUND DRAINS

Postoperative wound drains have been routinely placed for years following spinal surgery, to prevent buildup of blood in the subfascial space and to help minimize the incidence of epidural hematomas. However, multiple studies have demonstrated that prophylactic closed suction drains do not seem to influence the incidence of symptomatic epidural hematoma. Several of the large retrospective case series have specifically looked at this issue, and they have found no protective effect.[8–10] In the cervical spine, Herrick and colleagues[29] performed a retrospective review of 1799 instrumented posterior cervical procedures done at 4 centers and found that suction drains did not lower incidence of symptomatic hematomas. Brown and Brookfield[30] performed a prospective randomized trial of 83 patients with multilevel lumbar surgeries who were randomized to have a drain placed or not, and they found no difference in hematoma or infection rate in the 2 groups. Payne similarly found no protective effect of prophylactic drains in single-level laminectomies, in a prospective randomized study.[31] Again, given the rarity of symptomatic epidural hematomas, these prospective studies likely are underpowered to detect a difference in incidence. However no

study, either retrospective or prospective, has definitively shown any beneficial effect of closed suction drains after spinal surgery.[32] In fact Parker and colleagues,[33] in their Cochrane database review, could not identify clear benefits for their use in any orthopedic procedures. It seems that while prophylactic drains certainly make theoretic sense, there is no real evidence that they play any significant role in preventing clinically significant epidural hematomas.

CLINICAL PRESENTATION AND DIAGNOSIS

Most commonly symptomatic postoperative epidural hematomas evolve and become symptomatic within the first 24 to 48 hours after surgery.[4] However, this is not always the case. Uribe[9] reported on a series of delayed epidural hematomas in which all patients developed symptoms after postoperative day 3. Similarly, Anno reported on a series of 14 postoperative epidural hematomas where almost half occurred in a delayed fashion, at a mean of 5 days postoperative. The authors could not identify any distinguishing clinical features of the delayed hematomas compared with the immediate ones.[34] Aono[12] also noted half of the lumbar hematomas in his series presented in a delayed fashion, after the removal of the subfascial suction drain. So the development of an epidural hematoma remains possible even several days after surgery. Certainly, if a surgery was marked by unusual bleeding, if a surgery was performed urgently in a patient on preoperative anticoagulation, or if pharmacologic anticoagulation is necessary after surgery, vigilance and observation for symptoms of epidural hematoma should be continued for several days beyond the normal 48 hour window.

The diagnosis of a symptomatic postoperative epidural hematoma requires a high index of suspicion and is made on the basis of a combination of clinical symptoms and confirmatory radiographic imaging. Because asymptomatic epidural hematomas are so common when patients are imaged in the acute postoperative period, it is important to correlate MRI findings with clinical signs and symptoms. In the classic presentation, patients first report a severe sudden increase in axial pain in the area of the surgical site, which is greater than normal and often out of proportion to the surgical procedure. Within hours, radicular symptoms (pain, numbness and tingling) develop in the extremities, followed shortly by motor and sensory deficits and urinary retention.[3] Motor deficit can range from mild weakness to a flaccid paralysis, depending on the anatomic region. Neurologic findings may appear as myelopathy or complete spinal cord injury when the hematoma occurs in the cervical or thoracic spine, whereas it may resemble a cauda equina syndrome when it occurs in the lumbar spine. This evolution of symptoms from sudden axial pain to motor deficits typically evolves over 3 to 6 hours but may take longer. This classic progression of axial symptoms followed by radicular symptoms followed by motor deficits and sphincter dysfunction is also not always observed, and patients may rapidly progress from axial pain to neurologic deficit.

When a hematoma is suspected based on clinical symptoms, an emergency MRI should be obtained. Occasionally, CT-myelogram is necessary when patients have MRI incompatible cardiac or cochlear implants. In conjunction with clinical symptoms, a confirmatory MRI showing severe thecal sac compression will help make the diagnosis of a symptomatic epidural hematoma. The MRI will show a convex shaped fluid collection leading to severe thecal sac compression and narrowing.[35] In the acute phase after surgery, this collection will be isointense on T1-weighted images and hyperintense on T2-weighted images (**Fig. 1**). Radcliff has developed MRI criteria to help distinguish hematoma from abscess and pseudomeningocele.[36] Again, while some degree of hematoma and thecal sac compression is normal, severe thecal sac compression is not. In theory, the differential diagnosis for new, progressive weakness in the early postoperative period includes tumor, infection (epidural abcess), epidural hematoma and disc herniation. However, in practice, the abrupt presentation of an epidural hematoma is fairly characteristic and should be straightforward to diagnose.

MRI should be viewed as a confirmatory test to demonstrate the presence of a compressive hematoma in a patient where the diagnosis is already suspected based on clinical symptoms. Sokolowski and colleagues[37] tried to quantify a critical degree of thecal sac compression. They analyzed postoperative MRI's in three groups of patients: (1) patients with asymptomatic postop hematoma, (2) patients with severe peri-incisional pain but no neurologic compromise, and (3) full-blown symptomatic epidural hematoma with cauda equina syndrome. They calculated a "critical ratio" of thecal sac cross-sectional area on postoperative images divided by the thecal sac cross-sectional area on preoperative images. They demonstrated that thecal sac compression became gradually worse in the three

groups, with critical ratio measuring 0.8 in the asymptomatic group, 0.5 in the peri-incisional pain group, and 0.2 in the cauda equina group. However, these ratios do not represent hard criteria and postoperative MRI can often be difficult to interpret, particularly when spinal instrumentation is present. Thus the postoperative MRI should be viewed as an additional data point in the work up of a patient with suspected epidural hematoma and should be carefully correlated with the patients' symptoms. No specific MRI findings or degree of compression are considered pathognomonic for a symptomatic compressive epidural hematoma.

TREATMENT

Once a symptomatic epidural hematoma has been diagnosed, and MRI obtained, the treatment is emergent evacuation of the hematoma, ideally within 6 to 12 hours. Generally, the prior skin incision can be used but may need to be extended to gain access to all areas of compression. Often, when the lumbodorsal fascia is incised, the hematoma will be found to be under pressure and will "gush" out. The MRI should be carefully checked to see if the epidural compression or hematoma extends proximal or distal in the epidural space, beyond the limits of the original laminectomy or discectomy. If it does, additional levels may require laminectomy. After evacuation and irrigation, the wound and operative field must be thoroughly inspected to try to identify the source of bleeding and eliminate it to prevent recurrence. Epidural veins which are still bleeding should undergo bipolar coagulation. Any brisk bone surface bleeding should be treated with bone wax or numerous commercially available hemostatic agents. Muscular bleeders, particularly small arteries, should be searched for and coagulated, both with and without self-retaining retractors in place, which will sometimes suppress bleeding from the muscle. The wound should then be closed over a subfascial drain. Although data for subfascial drain use in primary surgery does not show conclusive benefit, given that the patient has required return to OR for hematoma, closure over a drain would seem indicated. Either immediately before or after evacuation, routine coagulation labs should be drawn and sent, in the unusual event that the patient has developed a coagulopathy. If the hematoma occurred in the setting of chemoprophylaxis for thromboembolism, anticoagulants should be held temporarily until the need for them is reassessed in consultation with the medical team.

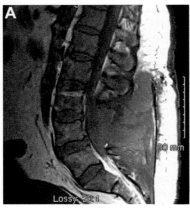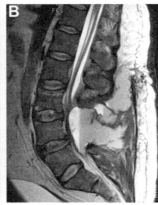

Fig. 1. MRI images of a patient who developed an epidural hematoma following administration of low-molecular-weight heparin for pulmonary embolism following lumbar surgery. (*A*) T1-weighted images demonstrate a convex mass, isointense to surrounding bone and CSF. (*B*) T2-weighted images show hyperintense mass with signal intensity similar to CSF, causing severe compression of the cauda equina.

OUTCOMES AND THE IMPORTANCE OF SURGICAL TIMING

The literature shows that by far the two most important prognostic factors which predict neurologic improvement after evacuation of epidural hematoma are the time delay to evacuation, and the degree of neurologic impairment before evacuation.[38] Once the diagnosis is made, evacuation of the clot should be carried out as soon as possible on an emergent basis. Several animal models of spinal cord compression have shown that duration of compression is a key determinant of ultimate neurologic recovery. Dimar and colleagues,[39] in an experimental rat model of incomplete spinal cord injury, applied spacers of varying size to compress the spinal cord of Sprague-Dawley rats for 0, 2, 6, 24, and 72 hours. He found that motor scores were consistently better the shorter the duration of spacer placement. They also found on histologic sections that histologic spinal cord damage increased as time of compression increased. Tarlov and colleagues[40–42] demonstrated similar findings in a dog model of spinal cord injury where an epidural balloon was used to compress the spinal cord. Again, recovery depended on force and duration of compression, as well as rapidity of onset of motor deficits. Delamarter also used a dog model of spinal cord compression and evaluated neurologic recovery following decompression immediately, after 1 hour, 6 hours, 24 hours, and 1 week. He found that with decompression immediately or after 1 hour, dogs regained ability to walk and recovered bowel and bladder control. When decompression occurred after 6 hours or later, no

neurologic recovery occurred and progressive necrosis of the spinal cord was seen on histology.[43]

Human clinical studies and case series of epidural hematomas have confirmed that severity of deficit and duration of compression are critical determinants of neurologic recovery. Lawton reviewed 30 epidural hematomas at Barrow Neurologic Institute and found that neurologic recovery was improved when evacuation was carried out before 12 hours. Eighty-three percent of Frankel Grade D patients improved compared with 25% of Frankel Grade A patients.[44] Kao also found a correlation between neurologic recovery and time to evacuation. In their series of 25 lumbar hematomas, they found that patients who had a complete neurologic recovery averaged 7.4 hours of symptoms prior to evacuation, compared to 17.9 hours in those with residual deficits.[14] Uribe was able to diagnose and evacuate all seven patients in his series within 6 hours, and 5 of 7 made a complete recovery.[9] Mukerji and Todd[38] in their systematic review concluded that operative intervention within 12 hours of onset of symptoms gave the best chance for recovery to normal. Incomplete deficits had better recovery than complete deficits in their study as well. Although no critical threshold can be discerned from human studies, it seems that neurologic recovery from epidural hematoma is maximized when neurologic deficits occur gradually, are incomplete, and when surgical evacuation is undertaken within 6 to 12 hours. Certainly, once the diagnosis of a symptomatic epidural hematoma is made, surgical evacuation should be undertaken as soon as possible, without delay.

SUMMARY

A symptomatic postoperative epidural hematoma is a rare complication of spine surgery, but if not recognized promptly, it can lead to permanent neurologic impairment and disability. Risk factors have varied in the literature, but include age, multilevel compression, and preoperative or postoperative coagulopathy. Making the diagnosis of a symptomatic epidural hematoma requires a high index of suspicion and is based on clinical signs and symptoms, as well as radiographic findings. Symptoms usually progress from severe axial pain, to radicular symptoms followed by motor weakness and sphincter dysfunction. Emergency MRI should be obtained, and if it confirms a compressive hematoma, evacuation and decompression of the hematoma should be done as quickly as possible, ideally within 6 to 12 hours. Neurologic recovery depends on time to evacuation and the severity of the neurologic deficit.

CLINICS CARE POINTS

- Symptomatic postoperative epidural hematomas are rare, with an incidence of 0.10% to 0.69%.
- Risk factors have varied in the literature, but multiple studies have reported advanced age, preoperative or postoperative coagulopathy, and multilevel laminectomy as risk factors for hematoma.
- The role of pharmacologic anticoagulation after spine surgery remains unclear, but multiple studies suggest it can be done safely with a low risk of epidural hematoma.
- Prophylactic suction drains have not been found to lower hematoma incidence.
- Most symptomatic postoperative epidural hematomas present within the first 24 to 48 hours after surgery but can present later.
- Diagnosis of a symptomatic hematoma requires correlation of clinical signs and symptoms with a compressive hematoma on MRI.
- Patients will usually first complain of a marked increase in axial pain, followed by radicular symptoms in the extremities, followed by motor weakness and sphincter dysfunction.
- An MRI should be obtained emergently, and if it confirms a compressive hematoma, surgical evacuation should be carried out as quickly as possible.
- The prognosis for neurologic improvement after evacuation depends on the time delay and the degree of neurologic impairment before evacuation.

DISCLOSURE

M. Djurasovic receives consulting fees and royalties for product development from Medtronic, consulting fees and royalties for product development from NuVasive, and Institutional Research support from Cerapedics, and Norton Healthcare. C. Campion has no conflicts of interest to disclose. J.R. Dimar receives consulting fees from Medtronic, consulting fees and royalties for product development from Stryker, consulting fees from DePuy, and Institutional Research Support from Norton Healthcare. S.D. Glassman receives consulting fees and royalties for product development from Medtronic, consulting fees from Stryker, and Institutional Research Support from Norton Healthcare, Intellirod Spine, Texas Scottish Rite Hospital, Alan L. and Jacqueline B. Stuart Spine Research Foundation, Medtronic, Scoliosis Research Society and Cerapedics. J. L. Gum receives consulting fees from Stryker, consulting fees and royalties for product development from Medtronic, Acuity, and NuVasive, and Institutional Research Support from Norton Healthcare, Texas Scottish Rite Hospital, Alan L. and Jacqueline B. Stuart Spine Research Foundation, Medtronic, Scoliosis Research Society and Cerapedics.

REFERENCES

1. Martin BI, Mirza SK, Spina N, et al. Trends in lumbar fusion procedure rates and associated hospital cost for degenerative spinal diseases in the United States., 2004 to 2015. Spine (Phila Pa 1976) 2019; 44(5):369–76.
2. Lambat MP, Glassman SD, Carreon LY. Impact of perioperative complications on clinical outcome scores in lumbar fusion surgery. J Neurosurg Spine 2013;18(3):265–8.
3. Al-Mutair A, Bednar DA. Spinal epidural hematoma. J Am Acad Orthop Surg 2010;18(8):494–502.
4. Schroeder GD, Kurd MF, Kepler CK, et al. Postoperative epidural hematomas in the lumbar spine. J Spinal Disord Tech 2015;28(9):313–8.
5. Glotzbecker MP, Bono CM, Wood KB, et al. Postoperative spinal epidural hematoma: a systematic review. Spine (Phila Pa 1976) 2010;35(10):E413–20.
6. Mirzai H, Eminoglu M, Orguc S, et al. Are drains useful for lumbar disc surgery? A prospective,

randomized clinical study. J Spinal Disord Tech 2006;19(3):171–7.

7. Sokolowski MJ, Garvey TA, Perl J, et al. Prospective study of postoperative lumbar epidural hematoma: incidence and risk factors. Spine (Phila Pa 1976) 2008;33(1):108–13.

8. Kou J, Fischgrund J, Biddinger A, et al. Risk factors for spinal epidural hematoma after spinal surgery. Spine (Phila Pa 1976) 2002;27(15):1670–3.

9. Uribe J, Moza K, Jimenez O, et al. Delayed postoperative spinal epidural hematomas. Spine J 2003; 3(2):125–9.

10. Awad JN, Kebaish KM, Donigan J, et al. Analysis for the risk factors for the development of postoperative spinal epidural hematoma. J Bone Joint Surg Br 2005;87(9):1248–52.

11. Yi S, Yoon DH, Kim KN, et al. Postoperative spinal epidural hematoma: risk factor and clinical outcome. Yonsei Med J 2006;47:326–32.

12. Aono H, Ohwada T, Hosono N, et al. Incidence of postoperative symptomatic epidural hematoma in spinal decompression surgery. J Neurosurg Spine 2011;15(2):202–5.

13. Amiri AR, Fouyas IP, Cro S, et al. Postoperative spinal epidural hematoma (SEH): incidence, risk factors, onset, and management. Spine J 2013;13(2): 134–40.

14. Kao FC, Tsai TT, Chen LH, et al. Symptomatic epidural hematoma after lumbar decompression surgery. Eur Spine J 2015;24(2):348–57.

15. Knusel K, Du JY, Ren B, et al. Symptomatic epidural hematoma after elective posterior lumbar decompression: incidence, timing, risk factors, and associated complications. HSS J 2020;16(Suppl 2):230–7.

16. Masuda S, Fujibayashi S, Takemoto M, et al. Incidence and clinical features of postoperative symptomatic hematoma after spine surgery: a multicenter study of 45 patients. Spine Surg Relat Res 2020;4(2):130–4.

17. Hohenberger C, Zeman F, Hohne J, et al. Symptomatic postoperative spinal epidural hematoma after spinal decompression surgery: prevalence, risk factors, and functional outcome. J Neurol Surg A Cent Eur Neurosurg 2020;81(4):290–6.

18. Fujiwara Y, Manabe H, Izumi B, et al. The impact of hypertension on the occurrence of postoperative spinal epidural hematoma following sigle level microscopic posterior lumbar decompression surgery in a single institute. Eur Spine J 2017;26(10): 2606–15.

19. Yamada K, Abe Y, Satoh S, et al. Large increase in blood pressure after extubation and high body mass index elevate the risk of spinal epidural hematoma after spinal surgery. Spine (Phila Pa 1976) 2015;40(13):1046–52.

20. Geerts WH, Pineo GF, Heit JA, et al. Prevention of venous thromboembolism: the Seventh ACCP Conference on Antithrombotic and Thrombolytic Therapy. Chest 2004;126(3 Suppl):338S–400S.

21. Fineberg SJ, Oglesby M, Patel AA, et al. The incidence and mortality of thromboembolic events in lumbar spine surgery. Spine (Phila Pa 1976) 2013; 38(13):1154–9.

22. Cheng JS, Arnold PM, Anderson PA, et al. Anticoagulation risk in spine surgery. Spine (Phila Pa 1976) 2010;35(9 Suppl):S117–24.

23. Kepler CK, McKenzie J, Kreitz T, et al. Venous thromboembolism prophylaxis in spine surgery. J Am Acad Orthop Surg 2018;26(14):489–500.

24. Cox JB, Weaver KJ, Neal DW, et al. Decreased incidence of venous thromboembolism after spine surgery with early multimodal prophylaxis: clinical article. J Neurosurg Spine 2014;21(4):677–84.

25. Gerlach R, Raabe A, Beck J, et al. Postoperative nadroparin administration for prophylaxis of thromboembolic events is not associated with an increased risk of hemorrhage after spinal surgery. Eur Spine J 2004;13(1):9–13.

26. Voth D, Schwarz M, Hahn K, et al. Prevention of deep vein thrombosis in neurosurgical patients: a prospective double-blind comparison of two prophylactic regimen. Neurosurg Rev 1992;15(4):289–94.

27. Schizas C, Neumayer F, Kosmopoulos V, et al. Incidence and management of pulmonary embolism following spinal surgery occurring while under chemical thromboprophylaxis. Eur Spine J 2008; 17(7):970–4.

28. Rokito SE, Schwartz MC, Neuwirth MG, et al. Deep vein thrombosis after major reconstructive spinal surgery. Spine (Phila Pa 1976) 1996;21(7):853–8.

29. Herrick DB, Tanenbaum JE, Mankarious M, et al. The relationship between surgical site drains and reoperation for wound-related complications following posterior cervical spine surgery: a multicenter retrospective study. J Neurosurg Spine 2018;29(6):628–34.

30. Brown MD, Brookfield KFW. A randomized study of closed wound suction drainage for extensive lumbar spine surgery. Spine (Phila Pa 1976) 2004; 29(10):1066–8.

31. Payne DH, Fischgrund JS, Herkowitz HN, et al. Efficacy of closed wound suction drainage after single-level lumbar laminectomy. J Spinal Disord 1996; 9(5):401–3.

32. Feras W, Alzahrani M, Abduljabbar FH, et al. The outcome of using closed suction wound drains in patients undergoing lumbar spine surgery: a systematic review. Glob Spine J 2015;5(6):479–85.

33. Parker MJ, Livingstone V, Clifton R, et al. Closed suction surgical wound drainage after orthopaedic surgery. Cochrane Database Syst Rev 2007;(3):CD001825.

34. Anno M, Yamazaki T, Hara N, et al. The incidence, clinical features and a comparison between early

and delayed onset of postoperative spinal epidural hematoma. Spine (Phila Pa 1976) 2019;44(6):420–3.

35. Braun P, Kazmi K, Nogués-Meléndez P, et al. MRI findings in spinal subdural and epidural hematomas. Eur J Radiol 2007;64(1):119–25.

36. Radcliff KE, Morrison WB, Kepler C, et al. Distinguishing pseudomeningocele, epidural hematoma, and postoperative infection on postoperative MRI. Clin Spine Surg 2016;29(9):E471–4.

37. Sokolowski MJ, Garvey TA, Perl J II, et al. Postoperative epidural hematoma: does size really matter? Spine (Phila Pa 1976) 2008;33(1):114–9.

38. Mukerji N, Todd N. Spinal epidural hematoma; factors influencing outcome. Br J Neurosurg 2013; 27(6):712–7.

39. Dimar JR, Glassman SD, Raque GH, et al. The influence of spinal canal narrowing and timing of decompression on neurologic recovery after spinal cord contusion in a rat model. Spine (Phila Pa 1976) 1999;24(16):1623–33.

40. Tarlov IM, Klinger H, Vitale S. Spinal cord compression studies: I. Experimental techniques to produce acute and gradual compression. AMA Arch Neurol Psychiatry 1953;70(6):813–9.

41. Tarlov IM, Klinger H. Spinal cord compression studies: II. Time limits for recovery after acute compression in dogs. AMA Arch Neurol Psychiatry 1954;71(3):271–90.

42. Tarlov IM. Spinal cord compression studies: III. Time limits for recovery after gradual compression in dogs. AMA Arch Neurol Psychiatry 1954;71(5): 588–97.

43. Delamarter RB, Sherman J, Carr JB. Pathophysiology of spinal cord injury: recovery after immediate and delayed decompression. J Bone Joint Surg Am 1995;77(7):1042–9.

44. Lawton MT, Porter RW, Heiserman JE, et al. Surgical management of spinal epidural hematoma: relationship between surgical timing and neurological outcome. J Neurosurg 1995;83(1):1–7.

Moving?

Make sure your subscription moves with you!

To notify us of your new address, find your **Clinics Account Number** (located on your mailing label above your name), and contact customer service at:

Email: journalscustomerservice-usa@elsevier.com

800-654-2452 (subscribers in the U.S. & Canada)
314-447-8871 (subscribers outside of the U.S. & Canada)

Fax number: 314-447-8029

Elsevier Health Sciences Division
Subscription Customer Service
3251 Riverport Lane
Maryland Heights, MO 63043

*To ensure uninterrupted delivery of your subscription, please notify us at least 4 weeks in advance of move.

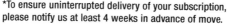